# therapy
# for
# stutterers

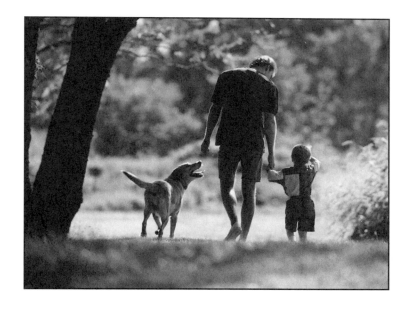

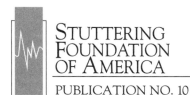

STUTTERING
FOUNDATION
OF AMERICA

PUBLICATION NO. 10

First Printing – 1974
Second Printing – 1984
Third Printing – 1989
Fourth Printing – 1992
Fifth Printing – 1996

*Published by*

*Stuttering Foundation of America*
*P.O. Box 11749*
*Memphis, Tennessee 38111-0749*

ISBN 0-933388-08-X

## To the Reader:

This book is written to help those who work or plan to work in therapy with adult and older adolescent stutterers.

The writers are speech pathologists who have specialized in the treatment of stuttering and are considered leading authorities in this field.

You will find their articles cover every phase of the therapy process and in so doing outline a program of treatment which we believe you will find effective.

All of the articles in this book were carefully reviewed, revised and approved for publication at a weeklong conference on the treatment of stuttering.

We hope that you can put this authoritative information to practical use in dealing with this baffling problem. Yours for effective therapy.

Jane Fraser

For the Stuttering Foundation of America
Memphis, Tennessee
January 1996

# Conferees and Authors

**Stanley H. Ainsworth, Ph.D., Chairman**
Alumni Foundation Distinguished Professor of Speech Correction, University of Georgia.

**Harold L. Luper, Ph.D.**
Professor and Head, Department of Audiology and Speech Pathology, University of Tennessee.

**Albert T. Murphy, Ph.D.**
Professor of Special Education, Boston University.

**David Prins, Ph.D.**
Professor, Programs in Speech Pathology and Audiology, University of Washington, Seattle.

**Harold B. Starbuck, Ph.D.**
Professor, Department of Speech Pathology and Audiology, State University College, Geneseo, New York.

**C. Woodruff Starkweather, Ph.D., Editor**
Professor, Department of Speech, Temple University.

**Charles Van Riper, Ph.D.**
Distinguished Professor and formerly Head, Department of Speech Pathology and Audiology, Western Michigan University.

**Dean Williams, Ph.D.**
Professor Emeritus, Speech Pathology and Audiology, University of Iowa.

**Malcolm Fraser**
Director, Stuttering Foundation of America.

# Foreword

As most of you know, adult stutterers are hard clients to work with for a number of reasons. When you first see them they're hard to evaluate. Later, they're hard to work with because their motivation may be low. When they are motivated, it's still hard to modify their behavior. Then, once their speech has improved, it's hard to keep it from slipping back into the old pattern. It's often difficult too for the clinician trained in speech pathology to cope with the shadowy world of the stutterer's attitudes and feelings. And finally, it's hard to work with adult stutterers because of the great demands therapy puts on the clinician personally.

We know the problems that you, the clinician, have in working with adult stutterers, and this book is an attempt to help you. For each of the areas mentioned above — evaluation, motivation, modification, attitudes, transfer, and the clinician himself, we have supplied a separate chapter, written by a speech pathologist who has encountered these problems many times. These authors have learned from their experiences and are passing on what they know to you in the hope that it will be a little easier for you and your clients to work together. Although it's the most exacting type of speech therapy, stuttering therapy is also the most satisfying, for the burdens of the adult stutterer are many indeed, and your assistance is welcome. The reward is in proportion to the challenge.

If you are familiar with some of the other books published by the Stuttering Foundation of America you will shortly realize that although this book bears some similarity to the other books, in other respects it is quite different. The differences result from the fact that it is a contemporary, updated description of how these authors are solving the clinical problems of the adult stutterer *now*. Moreover, they have sought to eschew theory and to concentrate instead upon being thoroughly practical. They have tried to put themselves in your shoes as you confront an adult stutterer and, from their long experience, they offer some clear illustrations of procedures for coping with his difficulties. They hope that the insights and suggestions will help you be a more effective clinician with adult stutterers.

C. WOODRUFF STARKWEATHER

# Table of Contents

*Foreword*
>C. Woodruff Starkweather ..................................7

*Evaluation*
>Dean Williams ...................................................9

*Motivation*
>David Prins .......................................................21
>Harold Starbuck ...............................................35

*Modification of Behavior*
>Charles Van Riper
>>Exploring the Problem ...............................45
>>Calming and Toughening the Stutterer............53
>>Modifying the Stuttering ...........................61

*Transfer and Maintenance*
>Harold L. Luper ..............................................75

*Feelings and Attitudes*
>Albert T. Murphy ...........................................87

*The Clinician and Therapy*
>Stanley H. Ainsworth ......................................105

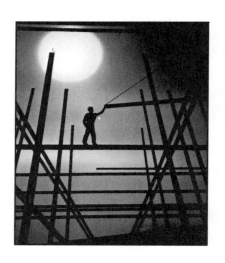

# Evaluation

There's no sharp division between the evaluation of a stutterer's communication problem and his program of therapy. When you begin your evaluation procedures, you're already beginning to do therapy. Conversely, as you start your therapy program, you're constantly evaluating, assessing, and reassessing those variables that seem to facilitate as well as interfere with progress in therapy. However, before you can plan a systematic program for the person sitting across from you, you first have to get a description of his stuttering behavior and then, insofar as you can, assess the effect that this manner of speaking has had, and is having, on his life. Keep in mind that all a clinician can do is help a stutterer learn how to learn to change his way of speaking, to change his emotional reactions toward himself and toward his listeners, and, most important, to adjust to those changes. Therefore, it's helpful to discover as much as you can about how he came to be the kind of person he is today — the beliefs he has, his attitudes about himself, and his perception of his relationships with other people to whom he has learned to respond with increased tension, concern, embarrassment, or withdrawal. These reaction patterns must be contrasted with attitudes and beliefs that create pride, strength, purpose, and happiness. To do this, it's helpful to explore both background and current information falling into five major areas: (1) case history; (2) description of speaking behavior; (3) variability of stuttering; (4) reactions to stuttering; and (5) personality factors.

## BACKGROUND INFORMATION

### Case History

Early in the evaluation you'll want to obtain a history of how the problem developed.

You have to be cautious, however, in accepting the stutterer's answers as fact. By the time he's an adult, many of the details of his younger years will have faded in memory, if in fact he ever knew them. This is true of information from a member of the family as well as that from the client.

Certain facts should be obtained because they will increase your understanding of the events that may have influenced or shaped the perceptions, attitudes, and reactions of the person as he grew older. This includes, for example, such data as the number of siblings in the family, the educational level of the client, etc.

Other kinds of information are helpful not so much because they're factual, but because they reflect the client's beliefs of "what occurred." Questions such as "When did your stuttering begin?" "What do you believe to be the cause of your stuttering?" "How did your playmates react to your stuttering?" etc. will bring out this information. These questions should be asked with the full realization that for any person, the things he believes are, for him, *facts.* A person operates and behaves as he *believes* things are in the world about him. If he believes something is true, he reacts to it as if it were "true." Therefore, it's important to get these statements from the client even though you know that they're his own or a member of his family's beliefs about what occurred and not necessarily the facts of the case as you perceive them. However, they are meaningful because they may be influencing his present day evaluations of how people react to him and how he feels about himself.

We aren't going to present a case history outline here. A variety of forms are presented in different textbooks, and most clinicians know where to find them. You may wonder which case history outline is the best, but there's no meaningful way to judge. Some are detailed. Others are fairly open ended. In some you simply "fill in the answers." You should become familiar with a variety of them so that you can devise a case history format with which you operate most comfortably. But you should never lose sight of the fact that when you're interviewing a specific person, you must not be bound by the apparent "inflexibility" imposed by the form. You have to be flexible enough to pursue any point that seems important. Study carefully the chapters in this book on motivation, therapy procedures, transfer and maintenance, etc., so you'll know just what it is you want to learn from the evaluation in order to develop the therapy program you want to use. Keep in mind that a question that may be irrelevant for one client should be pursued in detail for the next because it's of considerable importance to him. You should continually be asking, "Why am I asking this question?" For example, if a stutterer reports that he had a severe illness and was hospitalized for two weeks, why would you pursue this question and try to get more information? Is it because you believe there may be a direct relationship between the reported illness and the development or increase in severity of the stuttering problem? Or, are you concerned about when an illness occurred because of the effect it might have had on social activities or school achievement? Or do you want to find out about the effect it may have had on his attitudes and beliefs about himself and about how people treat him. It's your job to be sensitive to the significance a piece of information may have to the client's communication problem.

Any case history form is only a "beginning." The questions it lists are only representative. For example, "How did you get along with your brothers and sisters?" A thoughtful clinician could think about that question and then sit down and write fifty more questions that could be asked in relation to that one. As you get more experience, you'll realize more fully that a case history outline only guides the clinician into areas that need to be pursued.

With due awareness of the limitations discussed above, you'll want information about what may have affected the severity of stuttering, what may have increased the development of negative attitudes toward self and others. Sources for this information include: family history, educational history, social history, language and speech development, vocational history and future vocational plans, medical history, and stuttering history. Stuttering history is mentioned last because it can be pursued in relation to the facts obtained from the other areas. You'll want to know how these other variables affected, and were affected by, the development of stuttering. For example, under family history you might ask When did your parents report that you began to stutter? How did they react to it? What did they do to help? How did your brothers and sisters react to your speech and to you? The answers to these questions will provide information about the stutterer's perception, his *beliefs*, about their reactions to him as a person and as a stutterer. The same principle applies to the educational history. What educational level did he achieve? Was this influenced in any way by his stuttering problem? What kinds of grades did he receive? Does he believe that because of his stuttering his grades were lower or higher than they would have been if he hadn't stuttered? How does his school achievement correlate with any intelligence testing you might want to do? You'll be interested in his vocational plans to see if "what he wants to become in life," his goals, have been limited or facilitated by his stuttering problem.

You'll also want to know his beliefs about the nature of stuttering and what can be done about it. For example, you may want to find out what he believes is wrong or why he stutters. What has he done on his own in the past to "help" his stuttering? What has he found to be most helpful? What has he found to be least helpful? What does he do that he thinks might help but that results in his getting into "more trouble?" Tied to this, of course, is information about any previous therapy he's had. His attitudes and beliefs about previous therapy experiences will affect directly the way he responds to working with you. Therefore, you might want to ask such questions as, What previous therapy have you had? When? How long? What do you remember about what you did in therapy? Why do you think you did those things? How did you react to them? What was most helpful to you in therapy? Why? What was least helpful and what activities made no sense to you? Why? What have you learned from the therapy you've had? What do you believe would be helpful for you to do in therapy?

In addition to obtaining a history from the stutterer, we are interested, if possible, in finding out what the people who interact with him closely think about the problem. They may be his parents if he's living at home or has frequent contacts with them, or they may be a close friend or a spouse. In any event a comparison of how other people "see him" with how he "sees himself" is helpful.

A case history, then, is a way of bringing up to date the things that have influenced and are influencing the stutterer's concept of his problem. Remember though that anything that occurs, even one minute ago, is "history." As you become involved in therapy you'll still be interested in a "history" of his experiences from one session to the next. In this way you can help him evaluate and re-evaluate his social and self attitudes as they change along with his speech. These positive changes in attitude can be compared with those reported in his initial interview, so a fairly detailed case history can be helpful not only in planning therapy but also as a base from which to demonstrate improvement. Finally, the case history can be used as a vehicle for getting to know the client personally. Like any other form of interpersonal interaction, taking the case history is a structure through which you can form a relationship on which later therapy activities can rest.

## EVALUATION OF CURRENT STUTTERING PROBLEM

In therapy the stutterer changes his talking behavior so that it moves closer and closer to that of the normal speaker. Therefore, you'll want to assess whatever motoric reactions, emotional reactions, or attitudes and beliefs about speaking he has that interfere with moving in that direction. Some of the information gathered during this portion of the examination procedure will be related to information in the case history. For example, if your client was taught by a previous therapist to use a particular "stuttering pattern," you will want to find out if he is still using it partly or completely. Many other aspects of the case history will also tie in to the current problem. You'll want to look at his nonstuttered speech. Take a look at the rate, tension, and rhythm of speaking during nonstuttered as well as during stuttered elements. Think in time-space and get a description of the sequence of behavior. Does he, for example, speak with an extremely rapid rate and then slow down and begin to tense his neck muscles two or three words before he begins to "stutter?" Then, after saying the word, does he finish his statement on one exhalation with rapid rate and considerable tensing? This is the way to *describe* a behavioral sequence. You have to have a "then what does he *do* and then what does he *do*," way of observing. We are dealing with a behavioral *process*. It's helpful to learn how to describe it that way.

Speech can be described in several ways. First there are its audible characteristics. These include cessation of vocalization, part-word repetitions, prolongations, interjections, etc. Other dimensions include the tensing of muscles in various parts of the head, neck, and body, increasing or decreasing of rate of movement (speeding up of repetitions or interjections, etc.), and behaviors that are extraneous to talking, such as eye blinks, head jerks, etc. You should also describe any fairly consistent, steretoyped, patterns of behavior you see, such as interjecting a sound over and over and over until he says the following word with little or no difficulty. Or there may be a pattern of beginning to stutter and then backing up and saying two or three words, then beginning to stutter and then backing up again. One other common behavior pattern occurs when he begins to stutter overtly. See if there is a rapid acceleration of jaw movement and tension from the time when he begins until he completes the word.

A careful description of the behavior will provide you with vital clues for behavior modification.

Another dimension of speaking behavior is the "intent" or "purpose" of various behaviors observed. The evaluation of this dimension includes judgments on the part of the clinician which he'll verify through discussion with the client. Not only is the client helpful in assessing this aspect but in doing it, be becomes involved in his behavior in a way that will prove beneficial during therapy. Terms such as avoidance behavior, postponement, disguise, timers, starters, and holding back are judgments of the client's intent. For example, if you see him interjecting "ah" over and over for a period of time until the next word is spoken with no trouble, you might guess that the stutterer is using this as an "avoidance behavior." If he uses phrase repetition, i.e., when I, when I, when I gggo, you might guess that he's using the phrase to try to get a "running start" so as to "say the word without stuttering." The stutterer, upon reflection, can usually tell you if you're correct.

The two different kinds of information-gathering described above point out the importance of describing behavior in time sequence. When a "behavior checklist" is used, it's easy to miss the importance of what you're observing. For example, if a stutterer blinks his eyes rapidly, this information isn't too helpful by itself. But if he blinks his eyes rapidly just before he begins to stutter, then it may be that his eye-blinking is an attempt to avoid stuttering, or to "get the word out without any stuttering." On the other hand, if he has already begun stuttering and blinks his eyes rapidly in combination with a head jerk, then he may be using this combination to "help get out of the stutter." Therefore, many of the terms used by experienced clinicians to report speaking behavior involves not only descriptive but evaluative terms that ascribe an intent or purpose to the behavior.

### Variability of Stuttering

One feature of stuttering that is most confusing to the lay public is the extreme variability in frequency and duration of stuttering in different situations. You'll want to assess, as carefully as you can, the conditions under which the client's stuttering increases and decreases. Many clinicians have made up their own list of representative situations to use in determining the variability for any given client. These lists aren't hard to devise, if you don't have one, but many clinicians just use the ones they were given at graduate school. With a list, you can ask the client to rate each hypothetical situation on a five point scale with "one" representing little or no stuttering and "five" representing most severe stuttering. From this, you can devise a profile of the types of situations in which he has more difficulty and those in which he has less. The types of situations you might want to explore include (1) Increase in the number of listeners, — one listener, two listeners, small group, a classroom, a large audience, (2) The characteristics of the listener — women, men, persons older or younger than the stutterer, friends, strangers, boss, mother-in-law, (3) Nature of the speaking situation — asking questions, answering direct questions, telling jokes, giving short answers, explaining an event, giving directions, (4) The emotional setting — when he's in a subservient role, a dominating role, angry, embarrassed about an unrelated speech event, arguing, when he's not believed, when he's in the wrong and has to explain why, (5) Specific situations, phoning, making introductions — telling his own name, his address, his home town.

It's not only stuttering frequency and duration that vary from situation to situation. Emotional reactions vary too. You can use the same list of hypothetical situations described above to learn more about the variety of his emotional reactions in these situations. A five point scale can be used here too for him to rate the amount of emotional reaction. It's possible that in some situations he may report embarrassment, in others being ashamed, and in others being humiliated if he stutters. This presents an interesting dilemma about the concept of "severity." There are certain situations, such as arguing with friends, where the frequency and duration of stuttering may increase tremendously above a normal level but where feelings are not very intense. Conversely, while talking to the boss, he may avoid, substitute, and end up stuttering only one time, but the emotional reaction associated with that one instance of stuttering in front of the boss was extreme. These examples illustrate that "stuttering severity" is a multi-dimensional concept, and your evaluation will have to include all the dimensions, not just one.

Another dimension of stuttering variability is the *amount* of talking that is attempted. In some situations your client may volunteer a great deal of information, in others he may volunteer some, and in others little or none. There are other situations in which he'll talk only when he has to, and there are some that he will avoid entering at all costs. A profile of this aspect of his speaking behavior should be determined.

If you establish a situational profile of severity, emotional reactions, and amount of talking, this can be of assistance in two ways: (1) you can establish hierarchies of situations according to difficulty to aid in therapy planning and (2) you can use the profile information as a "base level" so the client can assess his improvement as therapy progresses.

## Reactions to Stuttering

Certain dimensions of the client's emotional reactions should be probed before you structure and plan a therapy program. An understanding of these reactions provides a perspective from which you and he can assess the emotional evaluations he's making as he talks in various situations.

Ask him what he's aware of when he's in the process of stuttering, what he's attending to. Is it other people's reactions, or his own "feelings," such as the hotness of his face, the lead in his stomach, the tightness of his throat. Is it the sound of his abnormal vocalization, or is it the "dead silence" of a silent block?

A similar question is "How do you think people feel about you or how do you feel about yourself when you stutter to them?" Does he think they feel sorry for him? Does he feel inferior to them? Does he feel childish? Does he feel that he'll be evaluated as not being "too smart?" Does he feel that whatever he has to say won't be considered important if he stutters while saying it? Will the person reject him and not want to talk with him if he stutters? All of these questions, and others that you can think of, will assist you in determining the direction counseling will take as your client begins to change his speaking behavior and to talk to more and more people.

You might also ask him what he does when he stutters, or is afraid he will do, that bothers him the most. Is it jerking his head? Is it running out of breath or a feeling of panic that he will run out of breath before he completes the word? Is it a fear that there will be no sound and he won't be able to move his jaw or mouth? Most stutterers have some aspect of their behavior that they dread much more than other aspects of it and knowing what it is can be a great help in planning therapy.

On the other hand, you should also find out what aspects of his stuttering bother him the least? What does he commonly do when he stutters that, if he didn't ever do any more than that, he wouldn't mind too much? Most stutterers will report, for example, that if they only had several part-word repetitions and that's all they did, they would be happy. It's when it goes beyond that point that scares him. By establishing a hierarchy of behavior fears, the clinician is guided in therapy planning.

A final dimension is what bothers him the most in listeners' reactions. Is he afraid that they'll laugh? Is he afraid that they'll give him a "sick smile?" Is he afraid they might interrupt him or look away or finish the word for him? Again, most stutterers fear certain kinds of listener reactions more than they fear others, and you should know what they are. This too can aid your planning.

## Personality Characteristics

During evaluation, the experienced clinician keeps asking himself, "what kind of a person is this?" He stays alert to cues in the client's general behavior from which he estimates how the client will react to him and to therapy. Is he the kind of person who will accept responsibility for changing what he is doing, or will he sit placidly by and wait for the clinician to do something "for him?" It has been said often that to be helped a person has to be helpable. There are certain ways of responding to people that either facilitate or hinder helpability. Many of these characteristics won't become evident until you ask the client to change some aspect of his behavior. The characteristics themselves are discussed in the chapter on motivation. During the first interview, however, you'll begin to make "guesses" about how the client will respond to therapy. Some hints can be found in the ways he has met problems in the past. In short, to what degree is he a "problem solver?" You'll need to know right from the beginning if you are going to encounter resistance or difficulties in motivating the client. As you take the case history and as the various speech tests are given, you can make observations and judgments about how the client has met problems in the past — academic problems, athletic competition, family squabbles, or dating problems. Is he independent, does he shift for himself in everyday life or does he wait for people to do things for him? As problems have arisen in the past, has he been action oriented, has he just talked about it, did he just wring his hands in despair? Does he want to know what *he* can do to talk better or does he just want to know what you can do for him?

Some clinicians like to have various personality inventories administered by persons qualified by training to give and to analyze them. The inventories are used to assess how personality characteristics might affect therapy. Again, however, use a lot of caution in evaluating what they "tell you." Personality inventories are best used by a clinician who ponders the responses and analyzes descriptively the possible impact of a client's score on, for example, a particular subtest of a personality inventory. This is much more helpful than just categorizing the client's behavior as either "abnormal" or "normal" on a particular characteristic. For example, the results of a personality inventory may indicate that the client is "highly anxious." Ordinarily, we're not as concerned about the fact that he may be "highly anxious" as we are about the way in which he uses the anxiety and what he's anxious about. We're all anxious to a degree, the point is whether we turn the anxiety inward and let it make our performance less effective or whether we turn in outward to help solve problems.

During the first interview, you'll be making some "first guesses" about characteristics that might interfere or facilitate the therapy process. Keep in mind that they are "first guesses" and be ready to modify and change your own evaluations as you come to know the stutterer better.

## PULLING THE INFORMATION TOGETHER

Although there are some clinicians who disagree, we think it's important to prepare a written report of your observations and impressions. It helps a clinician organize his thinking about the problem profile that the stutterer presents. It assists him in clarifying questions that he should have asked but didn't. It clarifies areas he should get more information about. It helps him think through the logical sequence for structuring an individual therapy program. Finally, it provides a structure from which the clinician can be alert to statements and attitudes the client may express as therapy progresses. If the written report doesn't do these things for you, then you shouldn't use it. The point is to find a vehicle which helps you rethink and integrate the information you have obtained, whatever form it takes.

You, as the clinician, must be versatile in implementing your therapy program to fit the strengths and weaknesses, the fears and self-confidence of the stutterer. We feel that the information described above will help you do it. Finally, we believe that the initial evaluation, if it's well done, demonstrates competence to the stutterer, it provides meaningful information for persons from related professions, and it provides a definable baseline for you and the stutterer from which improvements can begin.

DEAN WILLIAMS

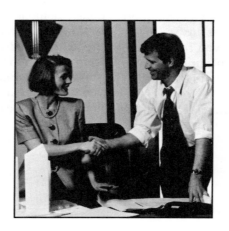

# Motivation

*part one*

"I came to see you because I'd like to do something about my stuttering problem." If a client begins this way you've got an excellent point of departure, for this is a statement of motivation. Motivation is the force that impels people to act. As one of the critical ingredients in successful treatment, motivation is something you have to be sensitive to. Properly directed, it provides energy that leads to change in therapy.

The source of high motivation are usually conditions that impel a person from within. For the stutterer, these include frustrations, fear, feelings of inadequacy, and the awareness that his speech deprives him of normal human relationships. These conditions bring about a positive desire to change.

Initially, there may also be factors that motivate the stutterer from without. These include coercion on the part of parents or a spouse, and peer group or vocational pressures. These are superficial forces, however, and if they aren't supported by an inner drive to achieve change, they will prove insufficient to sustain your client through the hardships of therapy.

At the outset you should realize that motivation is seldom maintained at a constant level. Your client will probably have a kind of motivational reservoir he can draw on, but its depth and clarity will vary with his changes in mood, the successes and failures of day-to-day experiences, his sense of progress, and the like. One of your jobs as a clinician is to recognize these changes and adapt your strategies to offset motivational swings. The continuing reappraisal of client motivation is actually a part of the on-going diagnosis that accompanies therapy.

Although motivation of the client will claim most of our attention, before proceeding further we ought to mention the *motivation of the clinician*. The confirmed stutterer brings to therapy perhaps the most baffling communicative disorder known. He may stop suddenly, fixate, re-treat, and struggle in an effort to produce speech. He undergoes severe social punishment as a consequence of this behavior, and yet at the same time he seems to possess the ability to speak normally. This paradox is one alley in a maze which has many obstructive pathways. As a result, therapy is often frustrating for you as well as the client. To help him discover the paths to recovery, you'll need first a thorough understanding of the problem and then intelligent planning, persistence, and the ability to suspend self-interest while investing your energy in the problem of your client. These are hard demands, in part because you're subject to swings in motivation as the stutterer is. Ultimately, your motivation is upheld, however by a fundamental concern for the individual, a desire to help him achieve more normal social relationships, and the confidence that you are able to do so. Your own motivation is actually one of the things that motivates the client. You can't depend on it to sustain him through therapy, but don't overlook its importance.

## RESISTANCE AND MOTIVATION

Any discussion of motivation brings up the matter of resistance. The two are often considered as opposite ends of a straight line. That is to say, high resistance leads to low motivation and vice versa. Though this simple relationship may apply to some clients, it doesn't apply to others. Let's look at some examples.

First of all, resistance is apparent when a client fails to cooperate in therapy or he tries directly to thwart it. Some resistance is inevitable. It results from the individual's natural reaction to change and his early efforts to test your competence. Consequently, you'll nearly always have some resistance to deal with whether motivation is high or low.

Consider the stutterer who begins therapy with high resistance. At first you may think his antagonism is just poor motivation, but as you help him understand his resistance, the energy he has used for this purpose can be converted to motivational force. In this way, a stutterer with high resistance may become a client with high motivation if you handle things well. If his resistance isn't resolved, however, you may be left with a client who offers only a weak effort to change.

Next consider the client who begins therapy with no apparent resistance. He's receptive, agreeable, and you're apt to think he's well motivated. Later you may discover that he's just apathetic about the problem or about the possibilities for therapy success. The absence of active resistance, then, doesn't necessarily foretell high motivation. In fact, it may mean just the opposite.

Of course, it may be your fortune to begin therapy with a highly motivated client with only mild resistance. Both of you are in just the right place at the right time. Therapy in this case has every opportunity to move smoothly and swiftly to accomplish the resolution of the problem.

In any event, one of your first tasks as you begin therapy is to recognize the characteristic signs of poor motivation and resistance, understand the dynamics behind them, and then adjust accordingly. These are the concerns of this chapter.

## SIGNS OF RESISTANCE AND POOR MOTIVATION

It would be nice if certain signs of resistance and poor motivation were always related to specific causes. Often, however, this isn't the case. A single cause may produce several different signs of resistance, or multiple causes for resistance may be revealed in a single sign. It depends mostly on the individual, and two examples will help to illustrate the point.

(1) A stutterer who doesn't understand the purpose of therapeutic procedures may show resistance by denying the problem, failing to accomplish assignments, and poor attendance. In this case, a single cause has produced

multiple resistance signs. (2) A stutterer who argues constantly could do so because he gets important secondary gains from his problems and also because he has a high degree of problem sensitivity. In this instance two sources of resistance produce one sign. In effect, the individual has a resistance "style" no matter what the cause.

With this background, let's look in more detail at some common signs of resistance and poor motivation.

### Arguing

Arguing is one of the most obvious signs of active resistance. From the beginning, some clients openly fight almost every suggestion and interpretation you offer. It's as if they size up the therapy relationship as one in which you're supposed to discover their faults while they're supposed to be clever and outwit you. As a result, you may be led into a fight to defend your ideas, and the therapy session can become an hour of conflict in which your insights serve only to challenge the client's debating skills. If you take this bait, you'll be more tired at the end of the session than your client. And you'll waste valuable time and end up in an adversary relationship with a person you're trying to help. There are times when disagreements have to be thrashed out, but getting drawn into debate

from the outset will impair your effectiveness severely. When a client does a lot of aruging, it's useful to keep in mind that he's actively involved, that he does have energy to pour into the task, and that this strength to fight back can be harnessed for therapeutic gain. With cases who argue, it's important to make them aware of what they're doing and explore the possible reasons. Some argument in therapy is natural and to be expected. A total absence might even be some cause for concern. But when arguing begins to consume time and energy, it debilitates the therapy process.

### Denying the Problem

More subtle than arguing is denial, or a refusal to accept the realities of stuttering. Though stuttering makes him miserable, a client may actually try to live as if it weren't there. For example, when a therapy group is first getting under way, some clients find a host of reasons why they shouldn't be involved in the group. Usually, they are stutterers with mild overt symptoms or who are successful in avoiding stuttering under certain circumstances. After being convinced that they won't catch a worse disease, and might even learn something in the bargain, they'll join the group. Then by direct statement or innuendo, they begin to suggest how much worse off the other group members are. Sometimes they aren't even willing to use the word "stutter" to describe their own behavior. This form of resistance is less directed at you than arguing and therefore may not be so easily identified. But it's poor motivation and resistance of the worst type. Denying the reality of the problem and being unable to accept an identity with others who stutter, foretell a major roadblock to problem resolution. The exploration and desensitization phases of your individual therapy sessions (see Van Riper's chapter in this book) will be helpful in combatting denial.

Group sessions can also be effective in coping with this form of resistance. Inevitably, other members of the group will react negatively to the person's attempts to place himself and his problems in a separate category. While this may cause him to be defensive for a time, appropriate exposure of his tactic in a group where there's mutual trust usually results in the breakdown of his defense and a gain of insight for him.

### Agreeing too Readily

When a client is utterly agreeable, you're not as likely to think about poor motivation as you do when faced with direct argument. Totally enamored with your suggestions, a client may seem completely pliable, bending without apparent resistance to the forces you exert. He goes along with your ideas and accepts without question what you have to say. He goes through the motions very well, but he may not be assuming responsibility for the outcome. He's not thinking, not questioning, not testing. In short, by doing what *you* suggest he is putting all the responsibility for the outcome of therapy on your shoulders. The poor motivation that produces this sign can be much more threatening to therapy success than motivational problems signified by direct argument and disagreeableness. You're more likely to recognize the latter as a sign of resistance, but the low motivational aspects of the former may only become apparent as you realize that little actual progress is being made. When a client uses agreeableness to resist accepting responsibility, it may be that he expects to fail and doesn't feel confident enough to risk self blame.

Because of its subtlety, this pattern of poor motivation is difficult to counteract in therapy. Often it becomes apparent when the client reports "I am trying everything *you* suggested, but *it* just isn't working." His language emphasizes your responsibility for the techniques you have recommended rather than an understanding that stuttering is something *he* does which he needs to change. This can give you a clue about what might be done. Help him think about the meaning of his words and refocus his attention on the exploration phase of therapy. He may then begin to see what he is doing and understand the problem in terms of his own behavior.

## The "Friend"

Sometimes a client is so engaging and witty that he disarms you with his pleasant personality. Gradually he becomes more like a conversational companion than a client. Then you suddenly realize that all you have to offer is companionship, which will probably be of little help in resolving the problem. When your client comes on like this, take a closer look. Is he saying, "If I make you my pal, you won't ask me to do unpleasant things or confront disagreeable ideas." This may happen when a person is afraid to discover the implications of his problem. He senses that he'll have to experience unpleasantness. He might even be afraid of some part of therapy. His light, superficial relationship with you might postpone or prevent these eventualities. As you recognize this, you can prevent a relationship from developing that will lack the character to work through the problem, and you can also be supportive of your client while assisting him in understanding his own behavior.

## Perennial Clients

Every now and again a stutterer will appear in your office who, in spite of rather severe speech difficulty, seems eager to talk and indifferent to the physical struggling that characterizes his speech. The longer he talks, however, the more you should be concerned by this indifference to speech difficulty. He may tell you about all the therapy he has had, that it has helped him some (his attitude is good now), and he wonders what is new on the therapy market. As he gradually becomes more absorbed in his history, he may regale you with stories about his problem, his therapists, and other fortunes of the speech war. You may begin to admire his equanimity, his ability to make the best of a bad situation and without consideration go ahead and sign him up for another tour of duty. Be careful. This may be a perennial client who has accepted all the wrong things about his problem and is living too comfortably with stuttering.

These characteristics are often seen in narcissistic individuals who find stuttering one of their most unique attributes. Though they suffer some frustration and embarrassment, they have come to enjoy the limelight that stuttering provides to an extent which offsets the negative aspects of the problem. They're inclined to be overbearing and may find themselves socially rejected. Therapy nicely fills this vacuum by providing a new group of enchanted listeners. The client's motivation in this case is to use therapy sessions to fill social needs. There's little chance for success unless this can be changed. By placing an emphasis on self-therapy and on the accomplishment of specific objectives, however, you can help determine the level of positive motivation. Then the clients who have little drive to change will either drop from therapy or face their weak motives and be helped to gain more positive ones.

## Poor Attendance

No matter what the behavior of the client during the therapy session, poor attendance is a frequent sign of motivation loss. There are, of course, reasonable excuses, but when they come often, it may be that therapy has a low priority. This is an easy sign to read, but you have to be careful to consider the reason. The client may simply have low motivation for any of the intrapersonal reasons we'll discuss in a moment. On the other hand, it may be that the therapy program itself is at fault and should be examined. It's been suggested that if absences, other than those for clearly unavoidable circumstances, exceed 15 per cent of the total possible attendance, then

something is wrong and corrective measures should be undertaken.

## Nonaccomplishment

The success of therapy usually depends a great deal on the amount of effort the client puts into self-therapy activities. In most therapy programs for older children and adults the client works on his own daily by entering speaking situations and by practicing and evaluating speech change. If your client continually "forgets" to complete these activities or makes other excuses, you may be sure that this important aspect of therapy is failing. If poor motivation is not a partial cause for this failure it will surely be an effect.

There are many reasons why a client fails to carry out these tasks. He may simply be afraid to risk change, or he may feel that what you've asked him to do doesn't make sense and that it won't help. He may fear failure, ridicule, or embarrassment. Any of the reasons for poor motivation can produce this sign. Some of these reasons will be explored in more detail in the section which follows.

## SOME CAUSES AND EFFECTS OF RESISTANCE AND POOR MOTIVATION

By the time a person has stuttered for ten years or more he'll have some very complex reasons for resistance and poor motivation. These will have been nurtured by his own personality, his home environment, his peer associations, his job, and his previous therapy experiences. As you come to understand these factors, you'll be in a better position to make adjustments in therapy to counteract them.

### The Raw Nerve of Stuttering

Stuttering can be a very sensitive subject. Both word and deed produce reactions by the stutterer and others which include embarrassment, fear, humiliation, and anger. As a therapist you want to take a close look at the problem, peel the protective layer from these feelings, and expose what may be the raw nerve of the disorder. When you do so, you'll re-expose your client to a number of negative experiences and the pain that accompanies them. The client often resists this. Not everyone who stutters reacts with this degree of sensitivity, but many do. The sources vary, but they are often found in early home experiences with parents who felt the problem was unacceptable and were ashamed of it and of their child. Severe ridi-

cule by peers during early school years is another source. But no matter what the cause, sensitivity is a compelling reason for resistance. If the behavior of stuttering is revolting or threatening to your client, he won't want to explore it or understand it, and this phase of therapy may be impaired.

### The Cure is Worse than the Disease

Many people who stutter do so infrequently. Even under stress, stuttering may occur on only two percent or less of the words spoken. When at ease, or having a good day, these people may not stutter at all. In many places, with some people, and much of the time, they pass as fluent speakers. They don't want to confront stuttering, they can't admit or won't accept responsibility for their behavior. These so-called mild stutterers often deny the problem. The hope that stuttering will simply go away has great appeal for them. The amount of fluency they enjoy is enough to keep the carrot of vanished stuttering almost within reach. In these cases avoidance motivation is strong, and it's fed and kept alive by the good chance that avoidance behavior will be successful. When you ask them to approach the problem, you're offering an unwelcome path. They feel that the cure, if it involves direct confrontation, is worse than the disease, at least in the beginning.

### The Feeling of Hopelessness

A history of therapy failure, particularly when accompanied by moderate to severe speech symptoms, can produce an attitude of resignation towards stuttering. Gains followed by relapse, or failure to make any progress at all, harden the stutterer to defeat. He has no real hope, and this prevents him from making an honest effort to take another step. His reason for poor motivation is actually quite rational. Based on the evidence he has seen, he predicts that his chances are poor. With the facts that he has at hand, this is perfectly true, and it's for this reason that ineffective therapy is so damaging. It's not only bad in itself, it lessens the chances of subsequent programs.

How does a person so defeated ever arrive at your door? Often he's pushed by family, friends, or employment considerations. Sometimes therapy has become almost a way of life. Even with no expectancy whatever that he'll improve, he comes to get some reassurance from the attention he receives when others show their concern for him.

### The Fear of Failure

The fear of failing is often strong in the adult stutter, and he may set up an excuse for failure in advance: "I really didn't go all out. It didn't mean that much to me at the time." He salvages some dignity by this fraud, and it leaves him some hope. Deluded by his rationalization, he keeps alive the notion that someday, if he really puts his shoulder to the wheel, he can do something about the way he talks.

This reason for poor motivation, which is present to some extent in almost all adult stutterers, prevents them from making a major breakthrough in therapy. To make real progress, a stutterer has to take risks. He risks the unknowns of listener reactions, embarrassment, discouragement, and even speech fluency itself. To do this requires self-confidence and the courage to face the possibility of failure with no one to blame but himself. This fear of failure can be one of therapy's immobilizers.

### The Removal of Self-Protective Responses

As currently understood by most clinicians, much of the abnormality in the adult stutterer's speech results from his attempts to avoid or escape perceived interruptions in speech flow. The avoidance-escape components of stuttering, which are a major target of most adult therapy programs, are instinctive, self-protective responses. We all flinch and draw back when signalled of impending pain. We all struggle to get away when we sense restraint. This is a matter of self preservation.

Stutterers therefore feel a strong need to hang on to their own methods of coping. Don't expect that your invitation to remove these responses will be met by immediate acceptance. When you urge the stutterer to touch his stuttering without recoiling, and to stutter smoothly without holding back, you are asking him to give up the very thing he believes has sustained him. You're attacking his solutions. He may try to change and do very well within the safety of therapy. But when the chips are down in the world he lives in, the self-protective responses will resurface almost automatically. There should be little wonder, then, that he resists giving up old patterns and exposing himself to presumed dangers, and that there is relapse under pressure.

With people who are hypersensitive to their own stuttering, who are dominated by hopelessness, who fear failure, or who can't give up the protective reactions of stuttering, it can be helpful to discuss these problems directly. By indicating that you understand these feelings and realize that under the circumstances they're reasonable, normal reactions, you'll provide support and the encouragement necessary to help them work through these

natural reasons for resistance.

### The Rejection of Change

"It may sound better to you, but it seems strange to me." Or, "This just isn't me talking. I feel silly talking this way." You won't need to work with very many stutterers before these comments become common. The stutterer usually rejects volitional responses which modify his stuttering or which increase his fluency. They're strange to his ear and to his kinesthetic sense. Like the organ transplant, these alien responses are rejected. Not only are the new ways of speaking physically different, but emotionally they may not fit the person's image of himself.

New ways of talking also make the stutterer feel conspicuous. As a child who says, "You can't see me," when he covers his eyes, the stutterer often believes that his ways of coping with the problem are unnoticeable. Also, at the instant he's caught up in the effort to avoid or escape, he may lose touch with what he's doing. In therapy when you ask him to do something that is highly volitional and noticeable to him and perhaps to his listeners, he'll balk. These changes will seem so clearly an improvement to you, that it's easy to forget that to the client they're physically and psychologically alien. Because of this, his motivation to accomplish speech change may be something less than you imagine. Part of therapy, then, is giving the client time to get used to change — to hear, see, and feel himself talking differently. It's useful to provide audio and video tape recordings for this purpose. By recording, playing back, and evaluating his speech in a variety of circumstances, the stutterer can gradually adapt to a new way of talking and a new image of himself as a speaker.

### The Need for Stuttering

One of the most often expressed reasons for low motivation and resistance is the secondary gain the client may get from stuttering. In the adult, this reason is of paramount importance. Anyone who lives for years with a socially handicapping condition, learns to use it to his advantage. He's only being expedient and there's no reason to suppose that the stutterer you're working with is any different.

Stuttering has many possible advantages. Most often it's a convenient excuse for failing to achieve almost anything. It's ego-saving to blame stuttering for vocational and educational failures, lack of friends, and poor relationships with the opposite sex. If your client has failed in these areas and has used this excuse, losing the problem may be a threat. It can be a sobering experience for a stutterer to consider how different life would be if tomorrow he didn't stutter. It's

often frightening for him to realize that he might be much the same person but without stuttering to fall back on.

There are other little advantages to stuttering, like the many ways it can be used as an excuse to keep from assuming reponsibilities. These are less serious deterents to motivation, however, than using it to explain life's failures. As a therapist, you face a major problem if your client is using his stuttering to explain his inadequacies. The problem is that his poor motivation from this source may not be immediately apparent in therapy since it probably won't produce any resistance on his part. It will become noticeable only later in a pattern of relapse and regression which so often plagues stuttering therapy.

Group explorations of the advantages of stuttering are helpful here. As group members begin to acknowledge some of the benefits of stuttering, the client may begin to see his reflection in the behavior of others.

### The Environment

Poor motivation can result from forces outside the stutterer, and you should be aware of them. With young people, it may be that a parent is sabotaging therapy. He may be openly negative about therapy, telling his son or daughter that it won't do any good and that it really isn't needed anyway. This can come from a parent who himself stutters and who has done little or nothing to resolve his own problem. A parent who feels guilty about his son or daughter's problem may also react this way. If he doesn't understand the objectives of the program or the nature of the problem, therapy will only highlight the problem and heighten his guilt feelings. Therapy to him is an admission that something is wrong and that outside help is required. It may increase frictions within the home that the problem has already caused. In the face of this kind of parental reaction, the client's incentive will be dashed, and he'll find it difficult to mobilize a wholehearted effort.

Reactions by friends can deter motivation. They may react negatively when the client fails to become fluent early in the program, or to changes the client is making in his speech. As he begins to avoid less and stutter more openly and smoothly, for example, they may object because the problem is more noticeable. This is particularly true of the mild stutterer who has been very successful in hiding his stuttering. If this situation prevails, it can dampen the ardor even of a client who has shown considerable enthusiasm about the changes he's making.

Vocational considerations can produce too much motivation. Employers who tell a stutterer that he must overcome the problem in order to keep his job may motivate him to a point of desperation. With such strong motivation to eliminate the problem, he may paint himself further into a corner. In spite of your honest efforts to have him reverse his avoidance-escape behavior, he may use the techniques of speech modification to further repress and to avoid. He will often experience temporary success only to have the effects of the technique wear thin as a result of its inappropriate use. Then, since he has been motivated all along to avoid, he quickly returns to former modes of behavior during stuttering.

## The Effects of Therapy Progress

One thing is certain about motivation — you should expect it to change from day to day. Although these changes may seem to vary almost at random, the reasons for them should be investigated.

For one thing, motivation can sag because of the progress a client has made. Signs of apathy appear, and he doesn't complete his self-therapy activities. Stuttering severity and frequency and speech fears are reduced, and this may diminish the incentive to continue working toward problem resolution. In other words, the payoff has been reduced and no longer seems worth the effort. If this happens, the client should be made aware that his reactions are reasonable, but he should also know that if vestiges remain of his old, reactive stuttering pattern, no matter how slight, they can be the seeds from which the problem will grow again. You can support his reactions but still give him the rationale for further effort.

### The Therapist and Therapy Program

When a client is poorly motivated or resistant, you'll probably want to blame him. But don't be too hasty. Take a hard look at your relationship with him and the nature of the therapy program you have developed. Other chapters in this book, and the rest of this chapter, suggest ways of relating to the client and ways to design therapy that will whet rather than damp motivation. You may be sure that if the adult stutterer doesn't know where he's going or why, if he doesn't see the sense of therapy procedures, if he can't see that progress is being made, his discouragement will mount and his motivation diminish.

With all of these reasons and with the forces of human nature apparently against motivation, what chance do you have? A very good one, actually, if you take steps to counteract the common reasons for poor motivation and if you're sensitive to your client's responses. Remember that his stuttering results in feelings of frustration, fear, and embarrassment. These produce discomfort and that makes him want to change. It's your job to capitalize on that drive.

DAVID PRINS

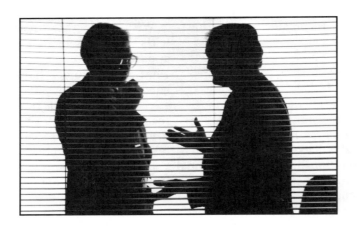

# *Motivation*

## *part two*

Now that we've discussed the causes and effects of low motivation and resistance, let's flip the coin and look at the other side. Let's look at some positive approaches and some solutions you might be able to fit into your therapeutic scheme. You understand, of course, that these are only suggestions, and you'll have to figure out whether you can apply them, or a variation of them, in your setting and be true to your therapeutic philosophy and style.

Motivation in therapy is an ever present consideration, and you have to be alert to capitalize on every opportunity, planned or unplanned. The first planned attempt to heighten motivation should take place when you meet your client.

## THE FIRST MEETING

Because the client has sought you out, you may safely assume that he's already motivated to work on his stuttering problem. The strength of this motivation, however, will vary, according to many factors.

One of the important determiners of motivation is therapeutic history, and particularly the number of clinicians the client has worked with. If you're the first, the client probably has high hopes and great expectations from a professional person after the many frustrations, false hopes, and failures of self-help, or the misguided advise of non-professionals who are functioning at the "folk lore" level. If this is the case, you're probably seeing a highly motivated person.

But if you're only one in a series of many professional clinicians the stutterer has seen, you'll probably have to overcome a resistance to therapy and a pessimistic feeling that nothing will help. Clients who have known failure before will expect it again, although they don't want to fail.

With such clients you should anticipate a low level of motivation and be forewarned.

It's important to note here that we said the stutterer has experienced failure before, not that the stutterer has failed. Too many times the failure is on the part of the clinician and not the stutterer. We are reminded of one boy, who, at the end of therapy said, "I'm going back to school and tell my speech teacher she didn't teach me nothing."

Hundreds of stutterers say the same thing when you ask them what their previous clinician had them do. They say that all they did was read from a book, read word lists, talk on a tape recorder, read poetry, or just talk. It is hard to put the blame on the client in such cases. You'll hear all kinds of stories, but if the person is still stuttering severely, you know that past procedures have not been effective.

Because your sole interest and obligation at the moment is the client in front of you, you must rapidly evaluate the accuracy of his reports and determine your next move. You won't want to blame anyone, but you should accept the fact that so far nothing has worked very well. This may be because his clinicians were inexperienced or not trained well enough, because the procedures they used were not the right ones for this client, because the timing of therapy wasn't right (the client wasn't "ready"), or because he wasn't motivated. Whatever you think the reason was, you want to absolve the client from blame, relieve any guilt feelings he might have, encourage him, and offer him hope that this time he may get help. You also want him to respect your knowledge and be motivated to make a new start with determination. Resistance is rarely encountered in early meetings, but by taking steps now you may prevent its appearance later.

You should make a good impression on any stutterer during your first meeting. Remember that he's evaluating you, just as you're evaluating him. He wants to know whether he's placing himself in competent hands. He'll have a good feeling toward you if you accept him as a person more than as a stutterer or client. Don't be outwardly concerned with his stuttering pattern until you actually begin your case study. The way you go about your job, the kind of things you say and how you say them, all affect his motivation. You can't underestimate the value of early rapport in establishing motivation.

## THE SPEECH EVALUATION

As you evaluate the client and his speech, use a clinical approach rather than an academic one. Ask your questions so that they relate to the client in front of you and his problem rather than to stutterers versus nonstutterers or to stutterers in general. There will be many opportunities later on in therapy to discuss such matters.

It's also good policy to lay out a few ground rules governing the evaluation and all following sessions. Explain to him that all discussions of his stuttering will be handled objectively, openly, and only as they relate to him and his problem. Stress your aim to be honest with him and that you expect him to be just as honest with you. Tell him that in your program you call a spade a spade, and a stutterer a stutterer. This should help the person who denies his stuttering face up to his problem. Some stutterers find great relief in finally admitting their stuttering exists and being able to talk about it openly and objectively. Don't use abstract terminology such as "dysrhythmia," "arhythmia," "covert stuttering," and "disfluency." These belong in the realm of academic exercise and have little place in a therapeutic workshop; they only confuse the stutterer.

In a similar vein, it's helpful to tell the stutterer that you have little clinical interest in the original cause of his stuttering, only in its correction. Tell him you must both look at the problem as it exists, and start your problem solving from that point. This may startle the perennial client (see Part I of this chapter), but it will tell him that you're interested in him and his problem. Discourage him from comparing your therapy with what he's had in the past.

Make your evaluation as efficient as possible. Know in advance what it is you want to learn about, and how to go about getting the information (see Williams' chapter of this book). Encourage him to speak openly and with no concern about his stuttering. Tell him you must see and hear it in order to evaluate it. Make comments or speculate on what you observe which show him that you know about stuttering. Be objective when probing a facet of his stuttering. Don't look too surprised and never act shocked or baffled by anything he says or does. Accept it as an everyday occurrence. Remember, he thinks you're the specialist. Be one.

If the client has had a lot of therapy before, it's a good idea to discuss it at this time. Ask him how frequently he was scheduled, how long each session was, what the therapy consisted of, whether or not he thought it helped him, and how he reacted to it and behaved in therapy. It's usually easy to explain previous therapy failure or limited success on one of the above points without demeaning the cli-

nician involved. Thus you have an opportunity to nip in the bud any resistance based on previous failure.

Many times the failure can be laid directly at the client's feet. This can usually be discovered from the way he answers questions about previous therapy. If you feel confident that previous failure resulted from his lack of activity, motivation, or involvement, the matter should be handled, immediately and objectively, in a firm and positive manner. Discuss with him the possibility that his previous failure resulted from his lack of participation. Explain why you think so and let him know that you won't allow the same thing to happen in your therapy program. You might want to explore with him the possibility that he has a "need" for stuttering and that he uses it as an excuse for failure. Judge his response to this and evaluate him as a therapy risk.

In some rare cases, it's best to refuse to schedule a stutterer for therapy. This should be done in a matter-of-fact way. Explain to him that you feel he's not ready for therapy, that his attitude toward therapy is poor, or that his presence in therapy might prevent other stutterers from achieving all they should. Tell him you're not going to waste your time or his if any of these things is the case. If he has a need for stuttering that's strong enough to preclude therapy success, counseling is the therapy of choice prior to speech therapy, and you should see that he gets to a competent professional.

If the stutterer is "testing" you to see how far you'll let him go in one way or another, you should set effective limits and stick with them. Doing so can turn his attitude from potential argument or sabotage to cooperation. This is another opportunity to let him know you mean business and expect the same from him. Keep all contact with him on a clinical level. There's no room for personal intimate friendship in a clinical situation. [Other clinicians feel exactly the opposite about this. See, for example, Murphy's chapter in this book. — *Ed*.].

On the other hand, if you have a very pessimistic client who has a strong fear of failure you must reassure him. Your problem is to redirect his thinking into therapeutic optimism. Be positive. Make it clear that temporary failures are an inevitable part of your therapy program. Assure him that you expect him to fail on some of his assignments, but in the same breath tell him you expect him to keep plugging away until he masters them and turns failures into successes. Note that his coming to you shows that he doesn't accept failure and is determined to keep looking for help and to keep trying. He's probably misinterpreted a lack of success as a failure. You'll help him regain his confidence by structuring early situations to assure early success and then working up to more difficult situations. Let him taste success and he'll want more.

## EARLY THERAPY SESSIONS

During your first therapy session you have a beautiful opportunity to motivate the client for all phases of the program. It's here, also, that many clinicians fail.

Many clinicians start out with a program designed to eliminate secondary characteristics or improve eye contact. The client, because of his initial motivation, usually works well at this and achieves good results. But as therapy goes on and the client sees no change in his stuttering frequency, he begins to wonder. He begins to doubt the therapy process, losing faith in you, and losing his motivation. Too many clinicians mistake "techniques" for "programs." They're adept at eliminating secondary characteristics or establishing eye contact, but beyond that they have no program. They then resort to reading from a book, or just talking about what the stutterer did over the weekend until he drops out of therapy.

The best way to prevent this from happening is to have a complete therapy program. By program we mean a total therapy rationale, organized in a sequence that will lead the client from where he is to being a fluent speaker. It's not enough to work just on secondary characteristics. You also have to work on the speech pattern, and you have to relate the speech pattern to the secondary characteristics.

If you don't have a complete program, prepare one. If you do have one, it's imperative that you explain it to the client during your first therapy session. You don't have to be specific, but you should present your program in a general way so that the client can evaluate it and see that it leads through a series of subgoals to his main goal. Let him know what lies ahead, and the amount of work he'll have to do. Explain aspects of your program that might not make immediate sense, such as working on eye contact, relating them directly to his speech. Explain why good eye contact is helpful and why poor eye contact is harmful. Outline your program so that he can see and understand that if he successfully completes each phase of it, he stands a good chance of attaining fluent speech. No client should have to work without knowing what he has to do and why he has to do it.

An explanation of the complete program serves as an ongoing motivational device. If the program is divided into phases or steps, accomplishing one phase motivates the client for the next. If your program is goal-oriented, these subgoals bring him one step closer to the main goal. The client who keeps missing sessions won't do so if he can be goal-oriented.

## LATER THERAPY SESSIONS AND REMOTIVATION

The old adage that success breeds success is as true in speech correction as it is in anything else. Very early in therapy you should introduce your client to others who have successfully participated in the program you outlined. This can be done in several ways. First, someone who has completed your program is your best salesman and motivational device. Have him show your client how he used to stutter. Let them discuss the therapy program, and many of your motivational problems should be solved. Second, a videotape of stutterers who have gone through your program is next best. Show them "before and after" tapes. The results should speak for themselves and should motivate your client to achieve comparable results. One advantage of videotape is that you can show a number of former clients with a variety of symptoms and severity. Third, an audiotape of speech samples is also pretty convincing and can motivate the client to work hard.

Don't ever forget that "results" is the name of the game, the stutterer's strongest desire, and our reason for existence. It's also the greatest motivational device, initial or ongoing, known. Show him some results and the client who's prone to argue will have little ground to stand on. Nobody can argue with results. Even if you can't produce instant results, your program should be sound enough, and you should be familiar enough with it to refute any argument with a reasonable and logical explanation.

By this time you should have established a high basic motivation, but you can't expect it to stay high forever. Stutterers, like everyone else, are subject to ups and downs, weaknesses and failures. Each new phase of your program will probably start off with a burst of enthusiasm and zeal. But once the subgoal is partially achieved you should expect a slackening of effort and drive.

The client will want to move on to the next phase, but you know he needs to master this step completely and strengthen his gains.

Now is the time to talk about failures. Tell your client what happened to so-and-so, who moved too fast through the program. Stress the need for overlearning and explain why incomplete mastery of one step can make it impossible to complete the next.

It might be wise at this time to play back the client's original recording. Let him hear how he once sounded, show him the improvement he has made and how far he still has to go. This should prove to be self-motivating, but you can help by itimizing the progress.

Another old adage is appropriate here. An ounce of prevention is worth a pound of cure. Don't let his motivation sag in the first place. You can prevent it by the way you make assignments. Be specific in identifying the subgoal the client is trying to achieve. Discuss how difficult the assignment is and describe some of the problems other clients have had and how they were resolved. Let your assignments be a challenge by telling him that many of your other clients have found them difficult. Encourage him to excel over the other stutterers you have worked with. Stress that you're asking for totally new behavior. Once again, don't let him work blind. Give him some suggestions about how to accomplish his subgoal. Tell him how others have done it. Let him participate freely in determining the details of the assignment. Predict how he'll do, and then see if he can match your prediction.

Be lavish with praise, but not indiscriminate. Praise any honest effort even if the desired results weren't totally obtained. When something is achieved, be sincere in your praise so he knows he's taken a step in the right direction. Use any accomplishment as motivation for strengthening past progress and as a challenge for the next.

You have to exercise a great deal of clinical judgment throughout therapy, but nowhere is it more critical than in determining when to move the client ahead from one step or phase to the next. Many clients get discouraged when they're kept on one phase too long. You have to watch out for this and sometimes you have to move a client ahead even though he hasn't reached your standards for subgoal achievement. You can always keep on working on a past phase of the program as you introduce a new one.

It should be inherent in your program that each step in built on the successful completion of earlier ones, and that subsequent steps include portions of preceding ones, so that the client is working on and strengthening previous gains as he works on a new phase.

## MOTIVATION BETWEEN THERAPY SESSIONS

Stuttering therapy hasn't received any outstanding achievement awards when it's done on a one hour per week or a half-hour twice a week basis. One of the reasons is that motivation may wane between sessions as the client gets interested in other events of his life. Many clinicians think that one of the greatest motivational problems is getting the client to work alone on his speech outside of formal therapy sessions. The spirit may be willing but the flesh is often weak. Some stutterers seem almost physically unable to propel themselves into a feared situation. A difficult job even when the clinician is along and urging and encouraging them, it's next to impossible when they're alone. You should schedule your clients for therapy as frequently as you possibly can, and then make it a point to see them on other days for encouragement. See them in the hallways, lunchroom, on the playground, anywhere.

One system that's been effective is the "buddy system." Depending on your particular situation, this "buddy" can be almost anybody. A good friend of the client, an employer, his girlfriend, a teacher, his wife, another stutterer, or anybody who shows a sincere interest in the client, his problems, and its management can be a "buddy." Most of all, it should be you, but when it's impossible for you to be available, have someone take your place. It's during these nontherapy periods that the client's buddy can encourage and motivate him to work or be a listener or critic. Goals can only be accomplished by hard and persistent work, and the client should be able to see that each successfully completed assignment brings him closer to his goals.

Naturally this will involve quite a lot of extra work on your part. You have to explain your program and techniques to the buddy, with emphasis on the immediate goal. He'll have to know what to look for, what to expect, what's good and what's bad. Have him sit in on therapy sessions occasionally to watch you and your techniques. Remember though that you're the clinician, and you should accompany him and help him work on his speech in real life situations as frequently as you can. You can plan the situation with the client and critique it later so that full value is received from each situation. This will also set a general pattern for all other situations the client does alone or with his buddy, and it will show him that you care about him and his progress, a strong motivational factor.

## GROUP MOTIVATION

In a group therapy situation, of course, you can divide the group into teams for speech work. This also requires considerable clinical judgment on your part. Select pairs that you think will work well together on the basis of personality, sex, age, accomplishment, severity, or motivation. Give them roles as clinician and client. Many times the slower achiever of the two, will work harder, longer, and better in the role of clinician while he's ex-

plaining a technique, demonstrating it, and correcting the faster client. He'll make progress in spite of himself. Many times also stutterers can accept criticism from other stutterers that they would reject from you.

Another effective technique is to divide the group temporarily into slow and fast halves without revealing the basis for your decision. Your reasoning will quickly be discovered, and the slow group will be strongly motivated to catch up. Then you can move individual stutterers from group to group and motivate them that way to either regain lost status or work harder to earn and retain a new status.

It's mandatory, of course, that you put the responsibility for speech correction directly on the shoulders of the stutterer. He must accept the fact that he's the stutterer, he has the problem, and he's the only person on earth who can work on his stuttering and learn to control it. You can give him knowledge, tell him and show him how to change his stuttering, but he's the one who has to do the actual changing. Impress upon him that he must learn to be his own clinician. Tell him that you can neither crawl into his mouth to manipulate his tongue, nor can you follow him around twelve hours a day reminding him to work on his speech. He must accept the fact that when therapy is over he'll be entirely on his own, and the quality of his speech will be in his own hands. Encourage him throughout therapy to take notes and gain as thorough a knowledge as possible about your techniques, your program, and the reasoning and logic behind them. Don't accept passive agreement and let him just go through the motions.

You can't be all things to all men, but at one time or another you'll find yourself playing the role of teacher, preacher, clown, father confessor, confidant, coach, mother, buddy, psychiatrist, counselor, disciplinarian, antagonist or protagonist, and clinician. All play a role in motivation at one time or another.

Punishment has been used as a motivational device, but it's usually effective only when it's constructive punishment. For example, if the client fails to complete an assignment, make him go back and repeat one that he's already completed before he can go on to the one he didn't carry out. This way you'll refresh and strengthen a previous aspect of therapy and then follow it by a successive step. This lets the client see the progressive nature of therapy, helps him enter a new phase, and it should motivate him to master it.

Motivation is something that must always be considered, and this includes *your* motivation as well as the client's. And how do you keep up your own motivation? By maintaining professionalism by attending meetings, workshops, and other sources of ongoing education and by reading your professional journals. Also by keeping your clinic or office an attractive and comfortable place to work in.

The motivation *you* have for your work will radiate to the client and will infuse in him a part of your enthusiasm and dedication.

HAROLD STARBUCK

# Modification of Behavior

## *part one*

### EXPLORING THE PROBLEM

So far we've been trying to help you understand the problems you'll encounter when you begin to help the stutterer overcome his communication difficulties. Now we come to the nitty-gritty of actual therapy. We'll try to tell you what to do, how to do it, when to do it, and why it should be done. Now this is, of course, an impossible set of goals. The uniqueness of each individual clinician and each stutterer prevents any specific recommendations from being universally applicable. Nevertheless, we can certainly give you enough basic guidelines and practical illustrations of therapy procedures to let you devise a therapy program for your client that's tailored to his special needs. We hope the activities we suggest will stimulate you to invent better ones, more appropriate ones. That being said, let's get started.

## How Should You Begin?

Stuttering often presents such a complicated picture that many clinicians aren't sure where or how to begin. We think we can help. In another book published by the Speech Foundation of America called *To the Stutterer* twenty-four speech pathologists, psychologists, and psychiatrists who themselves had been severe stutterers were asked to answer this question: "What advice would you give to a stutterer who, for one reason or another, can't get professional speech therapy?" Surprisingly, there were several things most of them agreed on, and one of these was that the stutterer should study his own stuttering. They expressed this in different ways but the emphasis was clear. If the confirmed stutterer remains unclear and confused about his behaviors and the feelings associated with them, his prognosis will be poor. This makes sense. The clinician's job is to facilitate learning and unlearning. If the client is to change his abnormal reactions to the anticipation or presence of fluency breaks, he has to learn what those reactions are. Also, when the client starts to explore his problem he looks closely at it, touches it, examines it, and often confronts it directly for the first time. He reverses the tendency to hide from it and to hide it from others. These confronta-tions are the beginning of desensi-tization. Therapy with the older stutterer should therefore begin with this confrontation and anal-ysis. There are some real advan-tages in beginning this way and we'll describe them later. But first, here are some examples of activities you might use.

Some of these suggestions will be inappropriate for certain clients. Some of them will be ap-propriate at one point in therapy but not at another. Too many clinicians feel uncertain about what they can do at this stage of therapy. That's because there's no way to get around the fact that each client has different needs, and his needs change throughout therapy. You'll have to use your clinical judgment about what procedures to use then, but here are some things you can do.

## Some Procedures

1. During the diagnostic exam-ination, provide a running com-mentary on what you observe the stutterer doing. 2. Demonstrate some of the anticipatory and re-lease reactions that you've seen in other stutterers and then ask your client to identify those that he too has experienced. 3. Play some audio or video recordings of other stutterers and have your client join you in their analysis.

4. Your client's own recordings can then be scrutinized in the same way. 5. Read and discuss descriptions from the literature on stuttering of the common feelings stutterer's have. 6. Before entering a feared situation, such as making a phone call or asking a stranger for directions, the client can write out or verbalize his expectations and feelings. 7. After he's entered feared situations try to express how you think your client felt and then ask him to correct any false impressions or, if you're lucky, you may be able to get him to describe what happened. 8. Tell your client you need to put his stuttering behaviors into your own mouth so you can understand them, and ask him to teach you how he stutters until your reproductions are fairly close. 9. Get him to collect samples of easy, unforced stutterings or to identify them in your own speech. 10. Have him say a stuttered word repeatedly to show him how his stuttering changes with adaptation. 11. From one of his recordings, have him count his stuttered and nonstuttered words so that he sees how much of his speech is fluent. 12. Use a stop watch to show him how long his stutterings really are. 13. Have him underline feared words before he reads a passage out loud, and then underline actual stutterings while listening to a recording of it; he may come to recognize the invalidity of some of his word fears. 14. Jointly make a catalog of the *variety* of his stuttering behaviors and then ask him about the purposes they may serve. (Why did he say "ah, ah, ah, ah," before that long prolongation on the /m/?) 15. Look with him for the presence of improper coarticulation in his repeated syllables; see if he used a schwa vowel rather than the vowel that should have been there. 16. Explore with him on videotape, or in front of a mirror, the abnormal mouth, jaw, or tongue postures he uses just before his speech attempt, comparing them with what he does when the word is spoken normally. 17. Explore his tremors, areas of tension, his avoidances, postponement, starter, and release behaviors. 18. Investigate with him his feelings of frustration, fear, shame, or hostility. 19. Determine the situational or phonemic or positional cues that trigger his fears of stuttering. 20. If possible, determine the vague outlines of his self-concept.

## Selecting Procedures

We've given a few of the many activities that can be used in this exploration phase. We're certain you can invent ones that are more appropriate for the specific stutterer you're working with. Also, we've listed these suggestions in random order. You'll have to arrange these confrontation experiences so your client won't be overwhelmed. Generally, you should begin with experiences that are least likely to produce resistance, anxiety, or other forms of emotional distress. Then you should sequence other exploratory activities according to his ability to tolerate or profit from them. Have him help you make these decisions. Have him rank a set of activities in the order of their threat, stress, or difficulty. Usually the client knows better than you what to confront first and what to postpone for later sessions. He may also be able to devise better experiences than you can. The important thing is to involve him immediately in the therapy process. He's not passive clay in your hands to be moulded to your liking. From the first, you should define his role as a cotherapist. He'll need some training first in how to be his own clinician, but both of you know you can't be with him all the time and that most of the work of therapy will have to be performed and designed by him. Sooner or later he'll have to become fully his own clinician, so it's best to get started and introduce this role as soon as possible. You're a guide, not the Magical Monarch of Moo.

### Why Begin This Way?

Some clinicians jump into the thicket of stuttering by asking too much of their clients too soon. They forget how emotional the adult stutterer is about his stuttering. They forget the blind hate he has for it. They forget how often he's tried to ignore it, disguise it, or pretend it doesn't exist. When climbing a long ladder it's better to put a foot on the bottom rung than to try to leap to the top. It's wise, then, to begin by stimulating the client's curiosity about what goes on when he stutters or expects to. If you can get him really interested in exploring his problem, you'll find some real pay-offs. First, he'll reduce the amount of running away, and hiding, and disguising he does because he's reluctant to expose his stuttering. If he's going to explore his stuttering, he'll have to seek it out. To examine it, he must be temporarily willing to experience it. Second, by exploring his stuttering in the presence of a warmly interested clinician who is permissive and not threatening, his fears, frustration, and shame will begin to decrease. Third, the disorder itself will lose some of the mystery that surrounds it. Finally, because of these things, some stutterers will show an immediate reduction in the amount of stuttering they exhibit while others may stutter more frequently but less severely. But even if no immediate change occurs in the severity or frequency of the stuttering, some basic changes in your client's attitudes toward his disorder are probably taking place. He's always been mystified and terrified by his stuttering. Now, in the relative safety of the therapy room, with you as a companion, guide, and co-explorer, one who is objective and analytical, interested rather than rejecting, he can touch the untouchable and scrutinize the inscrutable. Rapport, that indispensible ingredient of all therapy, is achieved more easily in such an atmosphere.

### Ways of Confronting Stuttering

Your client may prefer to talk in generalities about his stuttering than to exhibit it. All right, let's do that talking after he's given you some specific samples that can be discussed. Here are some things you can do to get those samples. With most stutterers, we recommend beginning with the oral reading of a passage about some aspect of the disorder, and as soon as a moment of stuttering has occurred, you should first duplicate it and then ask the client to do so too, before either of you talk about it. Ask him to describe the feelings he had before, during, and after the speech attempt. Reflect these feelings and try to clarify them. Ask him why he did what he did. What purpose, if any, is

served by a head jerk or a sudden exhalation of air. Give him some possible explanations and have him choose from them or ask him to volunteer some explanations of his own. State your ideas as hypotheses not as certainties, as inferences that must be checked out and tested. Have him compare the abnormal mouth posture he started to say the word with to the posture he used when saying the word normally. What was he really afraid of, if he was afraid? Were there old memories of past difficulty on that particular word or sound? What are some possible explanations for his eye closing or looking away? Where did the tension begin and how did it spread? What happened just before the final utterance of the word? Though we phrase these in terms of questions, they're for your use, not his. In discussing behaviors with your client, try not to cross-examine him. Try instead to get him to volunteer this information and to be interested in it. Try also to get him to use descriptive rather than evaluative language in his analysis. These are just suggestions. You may find better ways of helping him to know what he's doing or feeling.

Although we've found it wise to begin with oral reading, we soon shift to the narrative monologue as the material from which samples of overt and covert stuttering behaviors can be procured.

Have him talk about himself, the people who play important roles in his life, and about his stuttering experiences. We often tape record these sessions and then play them back to the client so that bits of behavior or expressions of feeling can be identified and discussed. Don't succumb to the temptation to lecture your client. Try to get him to say what he thinks before you offer your own commentary, then play the sample again for checking or for revising. Then use a mirror (preferably a full length one) or a videotape recorder to aid in the objective scrutiny.

Next, we recommend that you use conversational dialogue as the vehicle for exploring, analyzing, and cataloging. The topics of the conversation should again be stuttering as a disorder, his own particular stuttering behaviors and the feelings associated with them, or the goals and processes of therapy. Often at this time you'll find him talking about his feelings about you. He may even do some testing to see if you're really competent or really committed to his welfare. Without being defensive, reflect these feelings as being entirely natural and show that you are interested and accepting. Though the ostensible purpose of all this exploration is to compile a catalog of the stutterer's common responses to the anticipation or occurrence of stuttering, you're also trying to build

a good working therapeutic relationship, and you're beginning to desensitize him at the same time. Additionally, you should use phone calls to provide samples for exploration. Or you can invite some friend or stranger to join you. The stress you produce this way may bring on stuttering responses you haven't seen before. Also, these situations may provide a useful transition to speaking situations in the outside world.

Since the world outside that therapy room is where the stutterer must do most of his living, we insist that, as soon as it seems appropriate, you and he get outside that room. If you don't make an effort to do so, you may never know how that stutterer really stutters, nor will he. As you know, stuttering can vary widely in its severity from one speaking situation to another. Ordering a cup of coffee in a restaurant, asking a bus driver a question, or asking for information at the airport, will bring on behaviors and feelings you could never have obtained through interviews in your office. You won't have to do much of this, but you certainly should do enough to get an impression of how valid his reports are. What's even more important, you'll be able to assess his strength so you won't overload him.

Perhaps most important, your willingness to share his outside problems, will help convince him that you're committed and dedicated to his welfare. Stutterers often doubt and mistrust their clinicians. If you're willing to go with him into feared situations, he won't feel so alone. Then too, after these outside experiences have been shared and discussed objectively in terms of the new information they provide, you'll have created a model of the sort of self-scrutiny you want him to do. If, in addition, you're also willing to enter another situation and duplicate the kind of stuttering your client has and then follow up with an objective analysis of what took place, he'll be tremendously impressed. Much of his resistance will disappear. Even one or two of these joint experiences can make a remarkable difference. From this time on, he'll not only be much more willing to explore on his own but you can also feel more confidence in what he reports as having occurred.

### When to End Exploration

We can't tell you when to end the exploratory phase. Only you can make that judgment, but here are some guidelines or goals. Can the client duplicate his stutterings with reasonable fidelity? Can he talk about their major features and dynamics? Can he discuss his feelings of anxiety, frustration, hostility, or shame? Has he brought, for your examination, trophy-samples of behaviors that have occurred outside the therapy room? Has he attained reasonable success in analyzing his behaviors during monologue, conversation, or on the telephone when you're with him? Has he become curious about and interested in what he does or feels when he expects or experiences stuttering? Has some of his testing and resistance declined? Does he value your companionship as a co-explorer? Is he becoming impatient to get on with the modification of the stuttering?

We know that these questions may be hard to answer but they are the guidelines most clinicians use in deciding when to move to the next phase of therapy, the desensitization phase. In making this decision, you shouldn't expect your stutterer to have accomplished anything. Though we begin with exploration, analysis, and identification, we keep using them throughout the rest of therapy as well. Over and over again the client will have to confront himself objectively. By beginning this way we make it easier.

CHARLES VAN RIPER

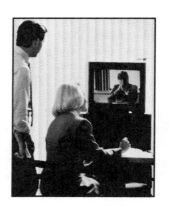

# Modification of Behavior

## *part two*

### CALMING AND TOUGHENING THE STUTTERER

Your next goal is to devise a program that will desensitize the stutterer to his stuttering. Some of this desensitization has already occurred during exploration and identification, but most stutterers also need intensive therapy focussed directly on cutting down their reactions to the expectations or actuality of stuttering. Great gains in fluency usually appear as they learn to calm themselves, but the big payoff comes later in the facilitation of new learning and unlearning they must do when they start to modify their stuttering behaviors. No stutterer can learn new ways of stuttering or better ways of living if he keeps getting bowled over by emotional reactions when he tries to talk. If you can toughen him to his stuttering; if you can help him learn that he doesn't have to panic when stuttering is threatened or experienced, progress will come more swiftly.

## How the Stutterer Feels

These emotions are mainly fear, shame, and frustration. As you know, stutterers fear certain speaking situations more than others, and they also fear certain words or sounds. These fears can be very strong, sometimes to the point of complete panic, and we must provide experiences that reduce their intensity and frequency. The stutterer's shame often shows up in his hesitancy to exhibit his disorder and in the many avoidance and disguise behaviors he uses to keep other people from recognizing him as a stutterer. Most stutterers find it hard to disclose these feelings of stigma except to someone they can really trust. Finally, you'll have to deal with your client's continual experiences of frustration. You mustn't ignore these feelings of frustration, for they may be even more important than the more evident feelings of fear and shame. Being unable to say what you want to, finding your breathing blocked, finding that you can't untangle your tongue, finding yourself mute, or realizing that you're hanging onto the same sound or syllable interminably when you want desperately to get on with your message is a devastating experience. When it happens hundreds of times a day, the cumulative frustration builds up until you can hardly keep from exploding. As a speech clinician, you've got to understand this frustration if you're going to help the stutterer.

So your job, in this phase of therapy, is to help the client learn how to increase his tolerance of communicative frustration, to reduce his feelings of shame and embarrassment, and to weaken his fears. How can you do it? There are several approaches and you'll have to decide, based on what you know of your client, which one or ones is best for his needs and capacities.

## Calming Him Down

Oddly enough, until a clinician helps them learn how, few stutterers ever try to calm themselves when confronted by the threat of stuttering. Yet, if a series of speaking situations is arranged in a hierarchy or ascending order of difficulty, and your client is asked to try to remain as calm as possible *while he's stuttering;* as he climbs each step of this therapeutic ladder, he'll discover to his surprise that he can control his emotions to a remarkable degree. The important ingredient in this kind of desensitization therapy is that your client must stay on each successive step of the hierarchy, trying repeatedly to remain calm, until he's finally successful. Then he goes on to the next step and does his speaking *and his stuttering* in this situation until again he finds success. The emphasis is not on being fluent in these graded speaking situations but in remaining fairly calm whether he stutters or not. Indeed, you should give strong approvals when your client does stutter yet shows no signs of emotional reaction and says that he felt pretty calm. There will be occasions when he won't seem to be able to stay calm. Don't accuse him of not trying hard enough. You've been pushing him too fast. You may need to revise the hierarchy by inserting some new substeps or rungs in the ladder of difficulty. There will also be times when your client will have to stay on one rung of that ladder for some time or even go back to an earlier step before he can progress. But sooner or later, if you're warm and approving when he makes some headway and reassuringly patient when he doesn't, he'll learn that it's possible to expect or experience stuttering without getting upset.

How long should your stutterer stay on one step before tackling the next most difficult speaking situation? We think he should keep on entering and re-entering the situation until he says and his behavior indicates that he has remained relatively calm during his stuttering moments. We can't describe exactly what the signs of calmness are, for they vary with each stutterer, but in general you'll find that the amount of forcing and struggling is lessened, the panicky avoidance and postponement and recoil behaviors are decreased, and he stutters more easily. His breathing is less disturbed. He says he's more calm. When these and other signs begin to appear with consistency, he's ready to tackle the next most difficult speaking situation in the hierarchy.

One of the best ways to help your client realize that it's possible to climb this ladder is to climb it yourself. You should do some pseudostuttering, especially on the early steps of the hierarchy, and show him that you can do so fairly calmly. Make sure you do this without offending the client, but do it. It's easier to touch a hot stove if someone else shows you he can touch it without getting burned. You'll be modelling a calm and objective attitude for your client. If you find it hard to provide this model, well, you'd better learn to desensitize yourself if you want to help stutterers.

## Testing Reality

Another important way to help the stutterer lose his speech anxiety and shame is to use the principle of deconfirmation. Most stutterers rarely examine those times when they expect a lot of difficulty but have little or none. All they remember are the times when their morbid expectations were confirmed. They'll tell you that they always have trouble, for example, on words beginning with the /p/ sound, or that they always stutter when talking on the telephone and so on. This isn't true, of course, but the stutterer believes it. Your job is to help him test reality. Help him get experiences in which he'll first predict the amount of difficulty he'll have in a speaking situation and then check, via tape recording or some other means, how often and how severely he actually stuttered. Or if he tells you that other people laugh at him when he stutters or that they show signs of impatience, or revulsion, again have him predict and then check. Over and over again, your stutterer will discover to his surprise that he rarely stutters as often or as severely as he expects to and that very few of his listeners really show the reactions he attributes to them.

### Eye Contact

Most stutterers base their expectations on just a few of their worst experiences (and there always are some, of course) but his usual expectations of evil are often exaggerated and even morbid. It's a good idea to give your client a chance to look closely and objectively at what happens when he stutters. This is why many speech clinicians work hard to get their clients to look at their listeners instead of lowering their gaze when they stutter or expect to. This habitual averting of the eyes during stuttering can be very

powerful and compulsive, and it's hard to change. The stutterer dreads the pity, rejection, impatience, or other reactions of his listeners, so he looks away. Unfortunately, if he keep doing so, his listeners will conclude that he's ashamed of his difficulties, and this makes things worse. By learning to look at his listeners while he's stuttering, your client can not only test the validity of his fears but also put his listeners at ease. Moreover, by maintaining eye contact the stutterer demonstrates that he's accepting, not rejecting, his stuttering as a problem to be solved. When he looks away he's denying the problem. It must be faced in the mirror of the listener's eyes.

### Self-Disclosure

The amount of energy most confirmed stutterers spend hiding their disorder is tremendous. They devise intricate strategies of avoidance and disguise. They assume masquerades of all sorts in the hope, usually a vain hope, that their listener won't recognize that they're stutterers. This burden is a heavy one and it only makes communication more difficult. You have to help your client stop pretending that he's a normal speaker and stop hiding the fact that occasionally he has some real difficulty talking. Help him experience the great relief that comes when he accepts his stuttering not as a miserable curse but as a problem that he's trying to solve. Now this doesn't mean that he should be willing to stutter but that he should be willing to show that he's working on his stuttering.

## Pseudostuttering or Faking

Another way of helping the client face up to his problem is by pseudostuttering, or, as it is sometimes called, faking. You can't just ask your stutterer to start doing it in all speaking situations. You have to first help him understand why it's useful and what the ultimate pay-off will be. You should plan for him to use it gradually and in a series of graded situations. You should be able to use some pseudostuttering yourself in speaking with him and in outside situations where he can watch you calmly exhibit stuttering as severe as his own. He'll see that most of your listeners don't penalize you. We suggest that at first you ask him to use pseudostuttering only on nonfeared words and that simple syllabic repetitions or fairly short prolongations should be the first kind to use. Again he should try to remain as calm as possible while exhibiting these voluntary disfluencies. Occasionally he should deliberately say the stuttered word again as though correcting himself, thus showing his listener that he's accepting his problem and working on it.

Later on, when he shows real progress in desensitization, the client should duplicate some of the features of his own habitual stuttering reactions. At this point, he may tell you that some of his faked stuttering turn into "real, uncontrollable stuttering blocks." This is an opportunity for you to tell him to try to keep the pseudostuttering entirely voluntary, even during the emotional reaction, and if he can he'll make great gains. He may have to pseudostutter more slowly, more deliberately, more strongly, more consciously, but he can learn that it's possible to maintain control. Once again, you should patiently clarify the reasons and goals for using pseudostuttering, and provide necessary approvals for progress. No desensitization procedure takes effect immediately; there are delays, slippage, and other fluctuations in progress. Through all this your client will need your support if he's going to learn that he can touch his stuttering, that he can deliberately put it into his mouth and exhibit it before strangers without having the skies fall down on his head. No one dies of a moment of stuttering, certainly not of a moment of pseudostuttering, but your clients have to learn to touch the untouchable and toughen themselves. By gradually learning to stutter on purpose and without pain, your client will lose a lot of the negative emotions that color his disorder; when this occurs, he'll find great relief.

### Tolerating Frustration

Much of the gross abnormality your stutterer shows is a reaction to his feeling that his utterance is being blockaded or that his syllables are recycling themselves out of his control. These abnormal reactions to communicative frustration have been learned, and they can be unlearned. No one has to stutter grotesquely, but your client probably won't have discovered this when he comes to you. His head jerks, gasps, and contorted features are usually reactions to frustration. It's immensely frustrating for him to open his mouth and find that he's mute. He'll tell you that it's a miserable experience to find his lips jammed together when he wants to open them, or to hear himself prolonging a yard of an /s/ sound when he knows that only a fraction of an inch of it is appropriate. By the time he comes to you, he may be automatically and involuntarily responding to these unpleasant frustrations with recoils, forcings, head jerks, or any number of other reactions that contribute to his audible or visible abnormality. Later on, you'll try to help him modify these behaviors, but at this phase of therapy your main job is to desensitize him to the frustration. If you can help him build up his tolerance to feeling blocked, he'll be able to bear his fixations or oscillations without instantly reacting in his old abnormal ways, and this is a great gain.

### Freezing

How can this tolerance to communicative frustration be learned? There are many ways of doing it, and you'll have to decide which ones are appropriate for the stutterer you're working with. One technique we've found useful is called freezing. Find a signal you can use the instant your client starts to prolong or repeat a sound or its posture. When he sees the signal he should freeze or immobilize his articulators (or continue to repeat the syllable if that's what he's doing), as long as your signal is being given. Make sure you have him hold the abnormality long enough to watch it in a hand mirror, or have it replayed on a delayed feedback apparatus or recorder, or while you duplicate it, or comment about it. Since the idea is to build up the stutterer's tolerance to the frustration and to prevent its triggering the recoil, forcing, or the other abnormal responses, you should gradually increase his freezing or holding so that he can tolerate more and more of it. Sometimes it's wise to have your client first give you the signal as you duplicate some of his characteristic behaviors, and when the signal is turned off, you should move forward into the rest of the word easily rather than using his characteristic responses. Make sure that he understands why he's doing what he's doing, that he must toughen himself to these frustrating stimili that trigger so much of his abnormality. Stutterers tend to go haywire when they feel blocked or reverberating and they do all sorts of maladaptive things that only make their problem more severe. If they can learn to touch the snake of stuttering without flinching, if they can make gains in tolerating communicative frustration, all sorts of good things happen.

### The Stuttering Bath

Another approach uses the principle of flooding. With a few especially courageous stutterers, a "bath of stuttering" can produce desensitization. The client is asked to collect a large number of moments of stuttering in a given time period or a large number of situations in which he stutters before he can go to bed or eat a meal. You can decide whether to accept pseudostutterings as fulfilling the quota at first, but it's best to insist on "real stutterings" as soon as possible. What usually happens is that the stutterer, for perhaps the first time in his life, wants to stutter, for each new instance of stuttering brings him closer to fulfilling his quota and getting reward or re-

lief. This approach isn't for all stutterers. Many would refuse or sabotage the assignment simply because they couldn't bear the experience. Nevertheless, if your stutterer can accept the challenge and does it to desensitize himself, the experience can produce some dramatic and favorable changes in his attitude toward his disorder and its treatment.

For most stutterers, the adaptation principle can be used. Have them repeat the stuttered word over and over again while trying to remain calm. There will be times when, after the word has been said fluently two or three times, the fear will build up again and more stuttering will result. You should try to arrange it so that he ends on a successful utterance and has signalled his feeling of calmness not only during the utterance of the word but in the stuttering period just prior to the attempt. Have him make a collection of some of the words he has stuttered on during the previous day and use these for adaptation practice.

There are other ways of decreasing the stutterer's fears, frustration, and shame. Some clinicians try to teach the stutterer to assume a state of deep relaxation while he imagines himself in a hierachy of feared speaking situations or as he attempts to speak. Some use strongly assertive and even aggressive behaviors to countercondition these negative emotions. Some use humor to counteract the fear or embarrassment. Some prefer to seek out and provide ventilation or resolution for the other anxieties or conflicts that augment the stutterer's communicative distress. Some feel that the stutterer will be less emotional if he examines his speech output realistically to determine the amount of fluent speech he already possesses. Most stutterers pay little attention to this fluent fraction of their speech output and tend to notice only the moments of abnormality. They often exaggerate and pump up their fears. By helping them look at their speech objectively, these clinicians hope that the stutterer will become less hypersensitive and morbid. All of us do all we can to build up our client's self-esteem and to reduce whatever seems to be lowering it, for we know that when his morale is high he's less vulnerable to stress and negative emotions. If we can help him solve some of his other problems, his problem of stuttering becomes more soluble.

Finally, we want to re-emphasize your role in this desensitization therapy. If you can accept his stuttering as a problem and if he finds in you a warm, trustworthy companion and guide, he too will come to acquire this attitude. As he exhibits his stuttering before you and finds that you don't penalize or reject him for it, his stuttering loses much of its evil emotional coloring. For once in his life he's found another person who understands how he feels and who's dedicated to his welfare. He's no longer alone. There's no better healing medicine than this.

CHARLES VAN RIPER

# Modification of Behavior

## part three

### MODIFYING THE STUTTERING

If your stutterer has made some real gains in identifying what he does when he expects to stutter or when he finds himself stuttering, and if he's found ways to stay calm during these episodes, he's ready to tackle a new set of goals. These concern the modification of his overt stuttering behaviors. Since the bulk of his abnormality usually consists of habitual responses to the expectation and experience of fluency breaks, your client will inevitably become more fluent if he unlearns them.

#### The First Goal

We have found it wise to begin by aiming our therapy at the reduction or elimination of the stutterer's avoidance and postponement responses to feared words and situations because these seem to be more under his control. Often they're used deliberately as well as automatically. Nevertheless, you should expect some resistance when these responses are attacked, and if you know why he resists giving up his avoiding and postponing, you won't be upset. For many years your client has been able to minimize his suffering by refusing to enter feared situations, by substituting easy words for hard ones, or by revising his sentences. By vigilantly scanning approaching speaking situations or prospective utterances, he has sometimes managed to escape the frustration or social penalties that otherwise might have occurred. Indeed, this avoidance has often been the only way he's found to reduce his distress. Avoidance responses can be very strong. You don't just tell him to stop avoiding. Even though he might like to or try to — and many stutterers hate themselves for always having to run away — at that last crucial moment of speech attempt, his old avoidance responses will dominate. And then he'll think of himself as a coward as well as a stutterer. He needs your help to eliminate them and he needs a systematic program to unlearn them.

What we've said about avoidance also holds true for postponement. The repeated use of an "ah" or an "um" or a "well, well, well-uh" just before attempting speech may be a large part of his abnormality, and it's clear that if these could be eliminated, much of his deviance would disappear. When he approaches a feared word, backs up, pauses, says previous words or phrases several times, it's obvious that these behaviors are impairing his over-all fluency and that he'd be better off if he didn't use them. Or perhaps he postpones saying the feared word by coming to a dead halt, a pause that not only breaks the flow of utterance but also produces frustration in the listener and the stutterer himself. Surely, you think, if he could eliminate these gaps in his speech, the stutterer would be more fluent. But these postponement behaviors have been very useful to him. Often they've helped him hide the fact that he stutters. Often, if he's been able to stall long enough before attempting a feared word or situation, he's discovered that indeed he didn't stutter. He'll ask you why this happens and you'd better have an answer. One explanation is simply this — fears, like other emotions, tend to fluctuate. They vary in intensity as time passes. At one moment the situation or word fear may be very intense; a moment later it may weaken. It flares and subsides like the flames in the fireplace. It rarely maintains itself at a peak level very long. The stutterer has simply discovered that, by postponing, he can sometimes manage to make the speech attempt at emotional ebb tide, at that fleeting instant when his word fear has declined almost to zero, and that when he can do so, little stuttering occurs. Yes, postponing occasionally keeps him from stuttering but the precision of timing is hard to achieve. More often than not, the very act of finally attempting the word causes the word fear to flare up again, and then he'll only have added the abnormality of his stalling to the stuttering it did not prevent. It's your job to help him realize vividly how rarely his avoidance, postponement, and disguise behaviors yield any real relief, and how often they contribute to the listener's impression of abnormality, how much they fracture his fluency, and how they actually reinforce his fears. Ducking and dodging and stalling and pretending are the things to be avoided — not the stuttering. If your stutterer is going to learn how to modify his stuttering, he simply has to come to grips with it.

### Stopping Avoidance

By now, you should have achieved a good therapeutic relationship and we hope your client prizes your approvals and is not indifferent to your disapprovals, for these are your major tools. They're the basic tools of every competent clinician. If you're operant-minded, you may want to devise an appropriate program that will decrease these behaviors.

If so, you'll have to outline it carefully, defining the behavior you want to decrease, deciding on scheduling, criteria, sequential steps, etc., and be prepared to do the necessary counting and plotting of responses. If operant conditioning isn't your bag, you still have to administer your approvals and disapprovals carefully, using them to facilitate your client's acceptance of the necessity to give up avoiding, postponing, and pretending he doesn't stutter. You'll use your approvals and disapprovals to help him become his own clinician with all the responsibility for planning and performance that this role requires. Help him devise and revise subgoals and strategies. Share your expectations and ease his hurt when he fails to corroborate them. We've had stutterers stop avoiding as soon as they realized that they were losing more than they gained from its use, but this insight rarely comes immediately or easily. Much of our effort is expended in creating conditions so that this insight can occur.

We now provide a list of some suggested experiences that have proved useful for most of the confirmed stutterers we've worked with. 1. During oral reading, ask your stutterer to try to use synonyms as substitutes for all words beginning with /p/ so that the garbling of his speech is made vivid to him. 2. Make a telephone call in his presence and, as you speak, duplicate the kinds of avoidances, postponements, and disguise tricks he uses. Discuss. 3. Engage him in conversation, and when he shows any of these behaviors, have him say the sentence they occured in twice over, duplicating the behaviors the first time, and then without them, before he can continue talking. 4. Using oral reading, have him rewrite the passage so that it includes all his characteristic avoidance, postponement, and disguise devices. You can use the format of the drama script with stage directions (*Look away and pretend to think here. Put hand over mouth*) to indicate the disguise responses. Have him help you design the passage. 5. Use a similar preparation for what he says when he makes a phone call. 6. Fill your own speech full of his characteristic avoidance, postponement, and disguise behaviors as you make a long phone call while he watches. 7. Using some recordings of his speech, have him identify and count how frequently these reactions were used and perhaps how long they lasted. 8. Analyze with him some appropriate recordings made by other stutterers so he can see how much of their speech abnormality was produced by the postponement and avoidances they used. Then scrutinize one of his own recordings from the same point of view. 9. Using a reading passage or prewritten sentences for paraphrasing or phone calls, have him load these excessively with the behaviors, then speak them over and over again *ad nauseum* until he's thoroughly sick of using them. 10. Devise a signal upon which he is to continue performing these behaviors until you signal again. Have your client use it on you first as you insert some postponement device of his into your own speech; then you apply it to him. Progressively increase the demand for continuation of the undesired behavior until it becomes distasteful.

## Reinforcement and Punishment

The activities described above are devoted primarily to building a vivid awareness of the behavior the stutterer should try to reduce, and to help him see that he should not be using it. We now suggest some other activities that use positive and negative reinforcement or mild punishment to decrease these responses. 1. Use the time-out procedure by insisting that your stutterer come to a dead halt and pause for five or ten seconds whenever one of these behaviors appears. 2. Turn your head away, shut your eyes, or cover your ears the moment you detect one of them in his speech. 3. Whenever he demonstrates one of them, duplicate it in your own speech or behavior simultaneously and continue it for a minute or so even as he continues talking.

4. Say "no, no" or give some other kind of disapproval whenever such a behavior occurs, then have him say it too when it appears. 5. Devise experiences in which your administered penalty or his own self-administered penalty is contingent on a certain quota of these reactions in a certain situation involving stress or during a certain period of talking time. Example: Have the client make ten phone calls before breakfast and postpone eating it (for a specified time) if he uses more than a certain number of word substitutions, etc. Have him select the time of the delay and set the number of word substitutions that would demand the penalty. 6. Have him signal each time he anticipates a feared word. Show him your approval when he says it without the old reactions. 7. After setting up a substantial quota of assigned oral reading time, paraphrasing, or phone calls, one that will ensure a considerable amount of labor and perhaps distress, reward him for each instance of direct attack on a signaled feared word by deducting a portion of that quota. For example, every time he refuses to substitute or postpone, the oral reading time is reduced by five minutes. 8. Have him stand on one leg until he has been able to read aloud for a set number of minutes without postponing. 9. With his help, devise a substantial reward for entering a certain

number of feared situations that normally he would have avoided. 10. For every speaking situation he confesses avoiding, have him devise an appropriate penance such as a certain amount of paraphrasing, oral reading, or phone calls.

Let's reiterate that these are just suggestions and that they may not be at all appropriate to the needs of the particular stutterer you're working with. They simply illustrate the kinds of things that could be done. As we've indicated, it's wise to have him help you plan the activities and set the performance quotas for the application of reinforcement or punishment. We structure the relationship as a co-therapist one. We work out these tasks and goals together, often setting maximum and minimum subgoals. We work hard to get the stutterer to administer his own approvals and disapprovals. When emotional reactions arise, we're there to help him weather them. A concerted attack on his avoidance, posponement, and disguise behaviors can't help but reduce them markedly, often to zero. Again, let's stress the need to achieve this reduction not only in the oral reading, monologue, and conversation that occur in the therapy room and in your presence but also in his everyday life.

## Fluent Stuttering

Your efforts to strip away the stutterer's defensive strategies for coping with his fears won't be effective unless you can offer something better to take their place. If he isn't going to avoid or postpone, *what is* he going to do? Your answer to this question should be very simple but direct: "Start saying the word you fear. Start saying its first sound. Start saying its first syllable. Sound out that word. Work through its motor sequence in a forward direction without interruption or recoil and do this slowly, deliberately, and strongly. Enter the speaking situations you formerly avoided, start talking and talk as much as you can and as often as you can. Instead of hiding and disguising the fact of your stuttering, display it openly but with this important difference — display it as a problem that you're obviously trying to solve." This is what the stutterer has to learn. These are the positive behaviors that you, as his clinician, must clarify and reinforce.

*When* should these goals be introduced? It's difficult to generalize, but usually we incorporate them after the stutterer has shown a fairly substantial reduction in the avoidance, postponement, and disguise behaviors. However, don't wait until they've entirely disappeared. Indeed they may not disappear until the stut-terer has made some progress in learning to approach his feared words and situations more directly and openly. You'll have to be the judge of this, of course, but you should know that it's possible to strengthen the new replacement behaviors at the same time that the old ones are being extinguished. You can, for example, give your approval whenever the stutterer begins a feared word by attempting its first sound even though he prolongs it and show your disapproval when he prefaces the attempt by "ah . . . ah . . . ah . . ."

*Where* should this work be done? Again, it's wise to begin in the comparative safety of the therapy room and in your presence. The stutterer will need you there to help him know why he should do what you're asking. There will be failures that you may need to interpret or assuage. You'll have to provide models of the behaviors desired. The stutterer will need your support and your information and your feedback. We suggest, as before, that the speaking of individually feared words, oral readings, monologue, conversation, and phone calls should be used as the vehicles of this new learning. We recommend that you accompany your client out into the real world a few times, enough times, to show him that he can function differently there too.

*How* can you help him learn

these new behaviors? If your basic orientation lies in operant conditioning, you can find examples of procedures and programs by Bruce Ryan and George Shames in another Speech Foundation of America publication, *Conditioning in Stuttering Therapy*, and we don't have to expand upon their contributions here. Instead, we'll present the rationale for the experiences we hope you can provide your client and then describe some of them.

There are a great many different kinds of stuttering behaviors. One stutterer shows one set of them; other stutterers show different sets. Even the stutterer you're now working with or planning to work with may stutter differently from time to time and it's almost certain that the variety of stuttering behaviors he shows now are unlike those he demonstrated when he was a child. Sometimes his struggling is very severe, but there are other instances when he seems to stutter easily. These easy effortless stutterings can be found occasionally in his speech and they're the goal models you should now try to set up for him. If he can always stutter in this easy way, the interruption to his speech flow will be minimal. These easy stutterings won't frustrate him and they won't frustrate his listener. He won't be penalized for them since they have little abnormaliy and so he'll feel no

shame. And he won't fear having to exhibit this kind of stuttering. If he can learn to stutter in this way, the vicious spiral can be unwound. If he can lose his fears, shame, and frustration, you can be sure that he won't stutter so often. By shaping the kind of stuttering he does so that it comes closer and closer to this model and finally reaches it, he can become a fluent speaker even though some residue of stuttering remains. At worst, he'll view his stuttering as a minor nuisance that he and others can easily tolerate; at best, he may attain the self-concept of being a mildly disfluent normal speaker and stop thinking of himself as a stutterer, for even normal speakers have their disfluencies too. You may ask, and the stutterer may ask you, if it's possible to learn to stutter in this new way. All we can say is that we've helped many to do so.

### Clarifying the Model

Your first task is to make it clear to the stutterer what it is he's supposed to learn. We've described the characteristics of this easy stuttering before but let's be more specific. The stutterer in attempting a feared word must try to begin it with the articulatory posture and movement that fits the first sound and syllable of that word when it's spoken normally. He shouldn't cock his mouth into an abnormal posture that might trigger a tremor. He shouldn't start it suddenly but as slowly as he can. Some stutterers who have learned it call this new kind of stuttering "slow-motion stuttering." He doesn't necessarily have to *talk* slowly but he should stutter slowly. The client should also learn how to make *strong* movements, not weak ones, but this doen't mean that he should abnormally tense his lips, tongue, etc. One stutterer said that he had discovered he could "stutter loose as a goose," whatever that means, probably that he no longer squeezed his lips or pressed his tongue or shut his ventricular folds tightly and then tried to blow the barriers open with a blast of air from a suddenly compressed chest. In this easy stuttering, most of the contacts are light, not squeezed firmly shut. Always, the movement is forward, the stutterer "sounding out" the successive phonemes sequentially. Once he begins the feared word, he doesn't stop; he keeps going — going forward in slow motion. The shifts from posture to posture are gradual, not sudden. No sound is elongated more than the others; all are slowed down proportionally. All this description is unduly detailed and you certainly don't need to explain it to the client. We might as well decribe how he should learn to skate. We provide it for your guidance, not his. Your job is to show him how to shape his stuttering so that it comes to resemble the new form.

As we've said, there are times when he already stutters this way and it really isn't a new way. If you have him say the same word over and over again, he will often be using the model a time or two before he becomes fluent. You can show him how to stutter this easy way by simply doing it and without any explanation at all. We've often taught young stutterers to do it by putting enough samples into our own mouth and then asking them to imitate us. Some stutterers have called it "the slide" or "the glide" or "sounding out." Most just call it "slow-motion stuttering" or "easy stuttering." What they are really doing, of course, is trying to say the word without avoidance or struggle. It really isn't necessary to stutter hard or abnormally.

*Activities for Easy Stuttering*

Now let's sketch a few of the many possible activities you might use to help him learn this easier way. 1. In your own speech, fake a few samples of your client's characteristic behaviors, then say the word again with the slow-motion, easy stuttering, then say it normally before proceeding. Have him "shadow" you, doing what you're doing as you say the word several times. 2. When he's talking and stuttering in his old way, repeatedly provide the model of the new form simultaneously with his stuttering. 3. Insert some duplications of his stuttering into your own speech and have him show you over and over again how you could use the new form as you continue your duplication. 4. Demonstrate one of his old abnormal trigger postures (lip protruding, etc.) and show him how to shift from this into a more normal beginning posture. 5. Have him assume one of these abnormal postures and change it several times back and forth into normal and abnormal positions before beginning the word. 6. Have him follow your model of shifting from tight lip or tongue contacts to light ones in the utterance of isolated feared words beginning with lip or lingual sounds in isolated words and then in sentences. Usually, when he adopts the tight contacts they will turn into tremors and he'll then feel that he's stuttering but this won't happen if the looser contacts are being produced. 7. On a feared word and especially one that begins with a vowel, you may notice that he shows a complete stoppage of airflow or phonation. This usually means that his ventricular folds (false vocal cords) are occluded. Most stutterers either recoil from this "blockage" experience and start over again or use an "ah" or inhalatory gasp or other means of opening the airway. There are better ways than these for opening that sphincter and one of them is to start with vocal fry and blend it into true phonation. Teach him to *search* for the adjustments he needs to make rather than to struggle blindly. 8. Provide your simultaneous modeling of a shift from high tensed oral musculatures into relaxed ones when he shows such marked tensions. 9. Reinforce with your approval all stutterings that are continuous rather than interrupted, all those that move forward even though at first certain sounds are abnormally prolonged but, as soon as you can, give him the idea that he should be making movements, strong ones but slow ones, as he works his way through the utterance of that word. Often the prolongation of the first sound of a stuttered word is only a disguised postponement behavior, the stutterer hanging onto it until the fear ebbs enough to decrease the probability of further stuttering. 10. Teach him to time the moment of speech attempt with a slow, strong jaw movement and help him know something about the appropriate co-articulation of the attempted syllable. Often the stutterer, consumed with fear of the initial sound, will be trying to say a syllable containing the schwa vowel rather than the vowel that's required. He tries to say the word "paper," for example, by producing the /p/ that belongs to the syllable "puh" rather than the right one. Sometimes you can help him get the proper co-articulation by having him pre-form the correct vowel in pantomime as he makes the speech attempt on the word.

We could provide many other suggested activities like this to help you solve some of the problems you may encounter but surely these will at least illustrate the general procedures. Your job is to start with the behaviors your client demonstrates and then modify and shape them until finally they approximate the goal behaviors. Often, to keep the model of easy stuttering before him, it's wise to ask the stutterer to fake frequently both the old and new forms on nonfeared words, thus providing the needed contrast. Sometimes it's wise to have him fill his speech with these easy slow-motion stutterings, saying all his words in this way for short periods to vivify the goal.

In this phase of therapy, then, the emphasis is on problem solving, on finding better ways of approaching and uttering the words he expects to stutter on. Your stutterer needs your observations and commentary if he's to make the necessary changes or even to discriminate what they should be. He'll also need your faith and support when temporary or partial failures occur. Some stutterers learn this better way of "stuttering" very easily; others need a lot of help and a lot of appropriate reinforcement. One way or another your job is to teach him that he can attempt his feared words without using the old avoidance and struggle reactions that constituted so much of his abnormality and disrupted fluency.

## Beginning Response Alteration

After your client has the model of new easy stuttering clearly in mind, and after he's had some vivid experiences in putting it into his mouth as well, we recommend that he use it in the process we've called cancellation. We refer to the practice of following each word on which the old forms of stuttering occur with an obvious pause and then repeating that word using the new form of easy stuttering on it before continuing. The sequence is 1. old form of stuttering; 2. definite pausing; 3. new form of stuttering. The cancellation in only a strategy you can use to help your client extinguish his old form of stuttering and strengthen the new. The pause functions as a mild punishment (time-out) but it also provides the time needed by the stutterer to help him identify what he did wrong and the time to make plans for demonstrating the contrasting new kind of stuttering when he says the word again. The latter, the new easy stuttering, must be done before the stutterer can continue speaking, so it's this that gets rewarded most strongly. Moreover, by using the cancelling process, the stutterer shows to himself and to the world that he's willing to work openly to change his abnormal way of speaking. And there are many other good reasons for using this strategy. You should at least explore its utility as a means of habituating the new easy way of stuttering. Even though the stutterer has shown you that he now has the capacity to stutter in this new way, this doesn't necessarily mean that he'll immediately be able to use it consistently wherever and whenever he wants to. Some of the old stuttering behaviors are bound to occur for some time. Cancellation can take care of them. Train your client to use it consistently in monologue, conversation, phone calls, and in outside speaking situations, both in your presence and when he's on his own.

### Better Reactions

Once your stutterer is willing and able to cancel his old abnormal responses and can do so with some consistency, it's wise to move toward their modification while they're still occurring. Show him how to release himself from his sticky, prolonged mouth postures or compulsive repetitions of a syllable in a less abnormal way. Perform his stuttering behaviors and then demonstrate better ways of releasing, of moving forward slowly and easily. Throw yourself into his characteristic fixations or tremors, then without stopping and trying again, loosen the tight contacts that he so often uses, get the air and sound flowing, and progress gradually from the sound to the correct syllable and through the utterance of the word. Do what he does when he stutters severely, then show him how to search for the correct articulatory posture, for the easing of hypertensed muscles, for the proper co-articulation of the syllable.

Often we've stuttered right along with our stutterers as they begin a moment of stuttering but then we release ourselves in better, less abnormal ways than those he's using. This stuttering in unison except for the better release you're demonstrating will soon teach your client to follow your example. Or you can assume his characteristic form of "blocking" and continue doing it until *he* shows *you* the kind of release you've been trying to teach him. Don't let him try and stop and then try again. Teach him to stay with his abnormality and work out of it in a more appropriate way. Help him modify his old stuttering patterns *while they're occurring* and reward all progressive approximations toward the easy, slow-motion, forward flowing response he's learned in the cancellation phase of therapy.

You needn't be alarmed if your client finds some initial difficulty in working out of his "blocks" in this new way. Reward the partial successes; clarify the goals; give him feedback so he can recognize not only what he's done wrong but also what he's done well. He's bound to get some partial successes if he keeps trying to change the way he usually responds to the experience of finding himself stuttering. For years he's just surrendered helplessly at these moments; now he's "wrestling with his demon" instead. Win or lose, it's a better feeling and a healthier one. When, for example, you find him beginning to say a /p/ word by protruding and squeezing his lips and then shifting to the new response of voluntarily retracting and loosening them before working through the rest of the word, you'll know that he's on his way. And so will he. Only a few experiences of this sort can make a tremendous difference. Though at first it may take a tremendous voluntary effort to resist the old manner of responding and to substitute the new, we've often been surprised to find how soon the latter becomes easy and automatic. Indeed there are some stutterers who learn it by themselves as soon as they've learned to cancel. It isn't necessary to struggle blindly when you feel yourself

stuttering. It's possible to stutter easily and with very little abnormality. There are thousands of ways of stuttering. Help your client find a better one. Many stutterers don't even call this way of talking "stuttering."

## Getting Set

There's no need for your client to cancel or wrestle with his stuttering for the rest of his life. If this were all we had to offer, the prospect would be a life sentence to hard labor and we wouldn't offer it. Fortunately it's possible to get set to say the feared word in the new way and then to say it in that new way. Many stutterers discover this by themselves; some need teaching. You may have to help him do some motor planning or rehearsing of the new easy stuttering before the speech attempt. Certainly you can clarify the model and provide the necessary challenge. Again, he'll occasionally get a few successes along with some failures and the former can be strongly reinforced. But what if he fails and finds himself in one of his old "blocks"? Well, then he can wrestle with it and modify it. And what if he doesn't do that either? Have him cancel it. And what if he doesn't even do that? Write down the word for him and have him use it again in another sentence some other time. Bind up his wounds and stay with him. The Rome of an easier way of stuttering isn't built in one therapy session. All therapy has its temporary failures. Progress never moves in a straight line. Though it oscillates back and forth it may still move forward. You'll find that as your client discovers the real fluency that comes when he can stutter easily rather than grotesquely any momentary set back won't matter much. Soon he'll be using the easier form of stuttering automatically and habitually and then he'll find it so much fun to talk you'll have to hide from him.

We've sketched the outline of one way you might help your stutterer to decrease his abnormality and increase his fluency. It's not the only way. It may not even be the right way for we can't know your client's personal characteristics, or his present stuttering behaviors, or his other personal problems. But far too many clinicians approach the responsibility for doing stuttering therapy with reluctance because they lack a comprehensive plan or because they have no rationale for what they do. If you're going to guide your stutterer out of the morass of his difficulties, you need to have some kind of a map. We've provided one for you. It's roughly drawn and not very detailed but it shows some of the routes both you and your stutterer might follow. Many have found fluency at the end of this trail.

CHARLES VAN RIPER

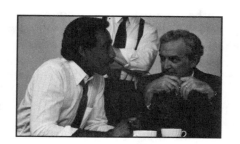

# Transfer and Maintenance

By the time your client has completed the programs outlined in the preceding chapters, he should be talking more fluently, coping better with his moments of stuttering, be less afraid of situations and words that used to throw him into disorganized panic, and be well on his way to acquiring a new self-image. It would be nice if you could at this point congratulate your client on his well-earned success and send him on his way. But there's still more to be done. Unless you take specific steps to ensure that the gains made so far are consolidated, the improvements in fluency and attitudes and the reduction of accessory behaviors may start to dwindle away as soon as frequent contacts with the clinician are ended. Unfortunately, stuttering seems particularly susceptible to recurrence. It's so common that the terms "regression" and "relapse" are frequently spoken by clinicians working with stutterers. And, as suggested in the chapter of this book by Prins and

Starbuck, unsuccessful therapy creates resistance and interferes with motivation.

Why is stuttering so tenacious? Why do the old behaviors tend to return after they've been modified or eliminated. There are many reasons. One of the most important facts is that stuttering isn't a condition like mumps where once the swelling is down it's gone. It's a complex set of highly integrated behaviors and attitudes learned under conditions of fear-avoidance and repeatedly, but intermittently, reinforced over a long period of time. Not only have the stutterer's responses been conditioned, but the cues or stimuli that lead to his anticipatory behaviors, tension, and escape devices have also been conditioned. Situations, words, listener reactions, even articulatory postures, can set off emotional reactions and coping behaviors. Let's look at some of these things in more detail.

## REASONS FOR RELAPSE

### Intermittent Reinforcement

Most of us are unaware of the powerful reinforcement in completing what we start to say. There's reward in saying what we have in mind. There's reward in positive listener reactions to our ideas. And there's reward in the feeling of "closure" to finishing the actions that are programmed in our brain as we start to speak. For the stutterer these rewards are even stronger because of the many frustrations he's had being unable to say what he wants to. So when a stutterer feels unable to say a word, he begins to search desperately for any device that will let him continue his utterance. When the "stuck" word is finally out, he feels relief from his frustration and a rewarding feeling for having completed his communication.

He's reinforced for anything he's tried in the effort to "free himself from feeling stuck" no matter how inappropriate. This happens hundreds of times a day for the average adult stutterer. And it's happened for years. No wonder his struggle behaviors are strongly learned.

But in addition to being powerful, the stutterer's reinforcements are also intermittent. It is a well-established fact that behaviors learned under intermittent reinforcement are more difficult to extinguish than those learned under continuous reinforcement. If a child gets a nickle every time he picks up his clothes for several weeks, and then suddenly the nickles stop coming for the same activity, he'll usually stop picking up his clothes after awhile. Once continuous reinforcement is removed the behavior soon stops. But, if the reinforcement is intermittent but frequent enough to continue a response, and especially if the child is never quite sure when he'll be rewarded, the behavior goes on long after the reward is terminated. Much of the reinforcement the stutterer receives is intermittent. Sometimes his avoidance behaviors get him out of the unpleasantness of being unable to continue his communication, but at other times, he still stutters. Sometimes when he jerks his head he's immediately able to complete the stuttered words, but many other times he can't. This intermittent, unpredictable reinforcement pattern makes the old stuttering responses very difficult to extinguish and very prone to reappear after they seem to have gone forever.

### The Difficulty of Extinguishing Avoidance Behaviors

Psychologists have long known that behaviors originally learned as ways of avoiding or escaping feared situations are particularly difficult to extinguish. Almost all stuttering behavior falls in this category. Attempts to avoid stuttering lead to much of the abnormal behavior. Again, these behaviors have been reinforced over and over again — but not predictably. The subtle postponement devices that many adult stutterers have get rewarded even

if they only delay the moment of unpleasantness temporarily. The fear of the stutterer is real. He's been stuck before, and he's had to endure negative social reactions from his listeners. He's felt what it's like to be unable to control his own behavior. And so anything that provides relief is strongly resistant to complete removal.

### Separation from the Clinician

By being a nonpunitive listener and by demonstrating that you could tolerate stuttering, your client's emotional and motoric behavior will have changed. Helpful as it is for you to have these characteristics during therapy, they can create problems after therapy is over. Your client's emotional reactions may climb when he realizes you're no longer around to support him and help him figure out what to do. Under this heightened emotion, his attempts to modify struggle behaviors may be unsuccessful. When this happens, it's not unusual for a client to panic and go back to his old avoidance or escape behaviors. Even if his stuttering behaviors don't return to their old severity and intensity, he may still have what has been called "failure trauma" — a frightening feeling that his temporary fluency was false and that he'll soon be re-experiencing all of the old fears and frustrations. To avoid this, you have to plan some specific measures to counteract it.

Separation from the therapist can also lead to regression because there is a change in rewards. During therapy, you've rewarded the client for activities he found difficult to carry out such as entering feared situations or staying with his difficult words until he found a more appropriate motor pattern. Few people outside the clinic will provide him with such rewards. They may still expect fluency and not realize that fluency is something you get by reducing old behaviors and learning new ones. They won't be around to say, "Hey, I was proud of you for speaking up in class when you were afraid you might stutter." Worse yet, they may reward the old pattern of doing everything possible to avoid stuttering. Under such conditions it's easy for the client to slip back into some of his old habits.

### Difficulty of Changing Self-Concept

Someone who's stuttered for years finds it difficult to think of himself as a fluent speaker or even a fluent stutterer. Subconciously, he can't fully enjoy his new fluency because of the recurring thought that his improved speech is just "false fluency." After all, he's had periods of fluency throughout his life, and they were always followed by renewed stuttering, so why should this change be permanent? Being fluent also brings responsibilities that can be difficult to accept. A fluent speaker is expected to participate verbally in group discussions, committee meetings, and bull sessions. The old self-image had a built-in excuse for avoiding such responsibilities. Sometimes the new self-image is hard to keep up because of the way friends and family react. They may dislike the personality changes that go along with fluency. The hesitant, cautious stutterer of the past rarely asserted his own feelings and opinions, and they don't know how to react now that he doesn't leave things up to them.

Some of your clients may find difficulty in maintaining their new self-image because of emotional rewards they got from their old roles. Secondary gains from being dependent on others, from having an excuse for failure, or even from listener punishment can cause resistance to change. Most of your clients will gain more than they lose by giving up stuttering, but the reasons for relapse are present often enough so that the possibility shouldn't be overlooked.

### Insufficient Practice

Normally the process of talking is a highly automated sequence of physiological activity. Muscle groups work in coordinated fashion to produce on-going speech. As some authorities have pointed out, stuttering can bring about deautomatization of these activities. Even a stutterer's fluent speech can be chopped up, hurried, or filled with frequent pauses and interjections. These "normal disfluencies" can sometimes precipitate stuttering. During therapy, your client has been learning to stutter in a more fluent way or to talk more fluently. Unless these new speaking behaviors have become automatic before therapy ends, your client may find it hard to maintain fluency under conditions of stress. Many authorities think that the main reason that stuttering reappears after therapy so often is that clinicians don't do enough to maintain newly acquired forms of fluency.

## COMBATTING REGRESSION AND RELAPSE

Regression and relapse don't have to occur. There are definite steps you can take to make sure that what your stutterer learns in the clinic will carry over to situations outside and will be retained after you stop seeing him. There are principles that help you know what to do to transfer a new behavior learned in one situation to other situations. There are also principles that help you plan how to *maintain* the client's newly learned behaviors over a long period of time.

The other chapters in this book give many suggestions about how to increase the probability that improvements will be permanent and widespread, but because stuttering puts up strong resistance to complete extinction, this chapter is devoted to the problems of transfer and maintenance. We feel strongly that any program of therapy for adult stutterers should include special attention to activities designed to solidify change after the client leaves your fold.

### Transfer Defined

The *transfer* of learning is the spread or generalization from the situation where the new behavior was originally learned to other situations or conditions. Although the term is seen most often in behaviorial modification literature, the concept is far from recent and is applicable to all therapeutic relationships. Many clinicians used to call transfer "carry-over."

Don't wait until therapy is almost over to start thinking about transfer. On the contrary, you incorporate activities designed to facilitate the transfer of learning right from the beginning and in every stage of therapy thereafter. For example, when you ask your client to explore and identify his stuttering behaviors, have him do some of his observation at home, in social situations, and at work, not just in the clinic and when he's learning to modify his stuttering, gradually lead him up to using his new behaviors outside the clinic. Of course you want to be fairly certain that the situations you ask him to enter don't create more anxiety than he can tolerate, since too strong a negative emotion may undo progress previously made.

The main principle to keep in mind is *stimulus generalization.* The more two situations are alike, the better chance your client has of transferring his new behaviors from one to the other.

Also, the greater the variety of situations he encounters with success, the more likely he is to be successful in *all* situations. With these principles in mind, you'll probably find it helpful to spend some time with your client discussing the many different situations he encounters, examining them for the amount of fear or speaking failure they produce, and then classifying them into groups of similarity. For example, one group might contain situations related to ordering items from sales people such as ordering meals in a restaurant, making purchases in a clothing store, or talking with a used car salesman about a potential purchase. Another group might center around talking to persons in authoritarian positions such as his employer, a teacher, a policeman,

etc. Once these lists are collected, you can start by role-playing the situations. Then ask your client to devise a plan for entering one situation from each group each day. Following the principle of systematic desensitization, he'll probably want to start with the least feared situations, first role-playing them in the clinic, and then entering them often enough to dissipate any residual anxiety before trying to enter the situations judged as next greatest in difficulty.

Often it's not possible to re-enter the same situation that has previously bothered the client. It is possible, however, to think of other situations that have most of the essential ingredients of the original and which can be entered. For example, a client who fears talking to an employer who's always critical of him can look for a local storekeeper who displays similar characteristics.

Here are some other ideas for activities you can use to see that transfer takes place. Have different listeners come in to the therapy room and talk with your client. Take him to a nearby classroom, a restaurant, a waiting room or any speaking situation similar to those he's likely to encounter in the future. Fortunately, you don't have to worry about running out of different speaking situations that will serve as good practice for the stutterer. Speech is an activity we use all day and every day, and almost any situation the client enters is a speech situation.

It usually helps for you to go with your client when you first send him out of the clinic for speech assignments. He'll need your objectivity in analyzing his behavior and the listener's response. You can also provide moral support by your presence, especially if you demonstrate that you can enter the same situations you expect him to and that you can be calm and unemotional in your own self-analysis. Gradually, you can wean him so that he takes the responsibility for his own selection of outside situations and for appraising his behavior afterwards. Retain some control over the outside assignments he selects however, so that you can gradually expand the range of speaking situations he successfully encounters.

Near the end of your formal therapy program, you can help him find a public speaking class to enroll in or a Toastmaster's Club to join. The importance of this type of activity is emphasized by the fact that 12 of the 24 recovered stutterers reported in a previous booklet (*To the Stutterer.* Memphis, Tenn.: Speech Foundation of America, 1973) that seeking additional speaking situations such as taking courses in public speaking, was a valuable part of their recovery.

The principles of fear reduction apply to feared words and speech sounds as well as situations. A stutterer may fear all consonants, all plosives, or even all words beginning with /s/. Practice in deliberately using his feared sounds until the fear is significantly reduced should help spread his newly developed feelings of confidence. Once the fear is reduced on one item such as words that start with /s/, other phonemes with similar phonetic characteristics, such as /sh/ or /z/ should be approached. In planning generalization activities, for words, it's wise to consider both phonetic and semantic similarity between words. For example, words pertaining to members of the family (*mother, father,* etc.) have semantic similarity, while words like *surf* and *serf* have phonetic similarity.

## Maintenance Defined

Maintenance means keeping the newly acquired behaviors going especially after contact with the clinician is discontinued. Everything you do in therapy is aimed toward the goal of maintenance, and if the earlier steps of therapy have been carried out appropriately, maintenance will follow automatically. Nevertheless, you should plan this termination phase of therapy just as carefully as the earlier stages.

## Suggestions for Maintaining New Behaviors

Prins and Starbuck, in their chapter of this book, stressed the need for a total program and for keeping the stutterer informed of the sequence and goals for each phase. It's also wise, toward the end of therapy, to call your client in and talk to him about the need and purposes of maintenance activities and about the differences in therapy at this stage. The main goal of this phase is a *shift of responsibility*. In the beginning, learning goes faster if you help the client identify his inappropriate behaviors and if you selectively reinforce ways of thinking and behaving. Eventually, however, the client has to assume this responsibility himself. Just as it's difficult for a teenager to become independent, shifting the responsibility for speaking behavior is also hard and is made easier if the shift takes place gradually.

How can you make certain that his new attitudes and behaviors stay with him when you're no longer around to reinforce or discourage? Here are a few suggestions. You'll probably think of others. You can plan a program to give him practice in being fluent. Many stutterers have developed habits of speaking disfluently even when not stuttering. They hesitate more, talk in shorter, choppier phrases, or even talk slower. Have the client try to maintain continuous, extemporaneous speech over periods of increasing length. Have him present memorized or printed material at increasingly rapid rates. A major aspect of therapy at this stage is the use of masking noise or delayed auditory feedback. The purpose of these techniques is to help him focus on the proprioceptive feel of fluency and away from the sound of his new speech pattern. You can find hundreds of ways to help him reach the point where fluency is automatic and much more than the absence of overt stuttering. Have him play the game of keeping a conversation going by rephrasing his conversational partner's last remark into a question, such as in Rogerian counselling.

Some clinicians have found that "heckling sessions" are useful, especially with a group of stutterers. Common communication disrupters, such as being interrupted, loss of the listener's attention, or demands for quick verbal responses can be used by the listeners, while the client has the job of staying calm and continuing to concentrate on his speaking behavior. If done properly, this type of practice can toughen the stutterer to resist similar communicative disrupters in the future.

Since most clients will probably revert at times to their old struggling behaviors, it's wise to include activities where they fake their old stuttering patterns and then follow up with appropriate modification. Role-playing situations in which the old stuttering returns but in which they react to it without panic can help prevent them from being thrown by such occurrences in the future. Faking such behaviors outside the clinic reinforces even more the substitution of responsible activity for guilt and dejection.

One of the most important aspects of this phase of therapy is preparing the client to resist reverting to old avoidance patterns. The tendency to use avoidances is established so strongly that they will return unless the client works diligently to prevent it. Especially if the stutterer has been experiencing a great deal of fluency, he'll find the tendency to use old avoidances very great when he feels any return of the old fear. Just as avoidances are the primary reason he originally developed all of his abnormal struggling behaviors, giving in to his avoidance tendencies can lead to their return. After long periods of fluency or successful coping, the first few times the client uses the quick little postponement devices they go almost unnoticed, but each use receives strong reinforcement for it prevents the overt return of the dreaded former pattern of struggling. Having been strongly learned in the past, these avoidances and postponement devices quickly return to full strength. Almost before the client realizes it, he's caught again in the old web of fear, avoidance, and struggle, but now there's a new dimension added. The return of the old pattern can bring feelings of guilt, hopelessness, and dejection.

Your terminal therapy program should therefore include some frank discussions about the part avoidance plays in the possible redevelopment of stuttering. It should also include some activities designed to resist this influence. You'll want to encourage the attitude that modification of stuttering behaviors is something he'll continue to work on after leaving you. Like weight-watching for the person who tends to overeat there are things one should and shouldn't do *from now on.*

### Developing a New Self-Concept

Activities in which the client has to practice maintaining the posture of a fluent speaker or in which he has to learn how to resist the attempts of old friends to force him back into his old role should be included in your terminal therapy program. You can also discuss with him some of the general characteristics of his past behavior to see if any of it may have been enhanced or resulted from his role as a stutterer. He may, for example, have developed a tendency to be hesitant and cautious in any speaking situation. Or he may have developed a pattern of concealing his feelings toward others in the same way he concealed his stuttering from his listeners. After analyzing these characteristics together, you can role-play new ways of behaving, focusing on general characteristics and not on his stuttering pattern. It often helps to have him experiment with different ways of behaving, rather than just trying to substitute a style that is opposite to his stuttering role. Some clinicians send their clients out into various situations, asking them to act differently — timid and shy talking to a clerk in one store, then aggressive and belligerent in the next. If the joint analysis you've done with your client indicates that certain people, like his father or mother, tend to reinforce his old self-image by the way they react to him, you can role-play the part of the family member while asking him to resist this influence.

## WHEN SHOULD THERAPY BE TERMINATED?

It's difficult to describe stutterers in the abstract, general sense and it's probably even harder to spell out when you should terminate your client. There are, however, several criteria. One is the obvious but difficult concept of fluency. Some clinicians set as their goal a certain percentage of stutterings or disfluencies. A few strive for zero stutterings. Others see this goal as unreasonable for some stutterers. Some clinicians state their goal in terms of fluency — distinguishing fluency from lack of stuttering — but including the concept of fluent stuttering as part of the end product of therapy. Some clinicians aim more for spontaneity and efficiency in communication and don't worry about some residual stuttering in the final product as long as the client speaks with ease and without abnormality.

We feel that the fluency criterion should be determined cojointly by the individual client and yourself. Together you should discuss the different expectations for fluency that he may expect to find looking at such things as the effects of different behaviors and the differences in the expectations of different listeners and in different situations. To use a broad generality, you should terminate your client when you feel relatively certain he can continue to improve on his own. There are signs that will help you know this. For example, your client should be coping well with the large majority of his disfluencies. The number of times his fixations and repetitions throw him into confused, random struggle behavior should be close to zero. And when this does happen he should be able to accept the responsibility for working on it. He should be able to analyze the problem and take steps to solve it. You'll want some reassurance that he can encounter pressures and threats to his new found fluency and self-image without yielding to them. Most important, his tendency to avoid should have been eliminated. Otherwise there would be a wedge to renewed development and maintenance of stuttering.

When the time for termination is imminent, it's wise to prepare him for the forthcoming separation. A session can be planned, in which you discuss his entire therapy program pointing out the times when he had difficulty, and reinforcing the many positive changes he's made. You'll probably want to make the separation gradual by reducing both the frequency of contacts and the degree of influence you exert on the topics of conversation. For example, instead of seeing him two or three times a week, arrange for "check-up" appointments at first weekly, then on alternate weeks, and finally stretching out to much greater intervals.

These check-up sessions are the basis for your *follow-up* program. As the frequency of the sessions decreases, give your client more responsibility for making written summaries of his progress, difficulties, and methods of coping. These written summaries are models for the reports you'll ask him to send you after all therapy contacts have been concluded. Have him also agree to keep you informed of address changes, and you might give him a supply of self-addressed postcards to be used at regular intervals. In our mobile, future-shock world of today, few people stay in one place very long. In asking him to give you follow-up information, tell him you want to find better ways to work with stutterers and that you're still interested in him.

In terminating therapy, it's always wise to set the tone so that the door is kept open for future contacts if he thinks they're necessary. Leave your client with the feeling that your concern is sincere and long-lasting. You don't expect him to need your help again, but if he does, you'll be there.

HAROLD LUPER

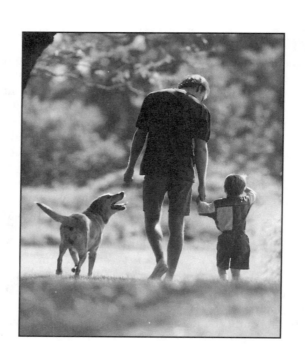

# Feelings and Attitudes

A five year old neighbor dropped into my study while I was working and asked why I had two pipes. I replied, "Oh, I guess to rest one while I smoke the other. Do you think a pipe needs to rest, too?" "No," he said, and I asked, "Why not?" He replied, "Because it's not alive." I asked him what "alive" meant, and he responded, "To be able to talk."

People who stutter would agree. Van Riper has said that stuttering isn't just a speech impairment; it's an impediment in social living. We would like to embellish that observation. More than a speech impairment, stuttering is a vast panorama, a series of dramas of the human condition. It is tragedy, farce, comedy. It is sad, wearisome, paradoxical, boring, clever, controlled, uncontrollable, sensitive, ugly. It has a cast of thousands, mostly male, but of all ages and all classes: kings, queens, composers, poets, thieves, scientists, patrons and peasants. It is everyman.

For some, stuttering is a way of life, self-destructive perhaps, but a way of life nonetheless. If this weren't usually so, if stuttering were only an imperfection in an otherwise healthy organism, the enormous difficulty most adults have in overcoming it would be hard to understand. Stuttering is often the hub of a complex system, generating its own goals and motivations, its own pains and pleasures. Often this system takes over large portions of the individual's capacities, consuming them for its own purposes. It is a system that feeds itself; it can grow and spread like a weed, and it's hard to uproot.

At the same time, stuttering is one way of being and becoming human. And although it is not the path most people take, it is well-traveled. It is more tortuous than most paths, and it can be rugged and painful. There are better paths to becoming most fully human. Your goal as a clinician is to help the stuttering person find better ways, ways to richer human existence through increased communicative effectiveness. When clinicians strive toward this goal, they widen their professional repertoire. Helping others to create and to recreate themselves, you may also find yourself in a process of personal renewal. Stuttering therapy can be a remarkable opportunity for you to become more fully human in relationship with others in need.

Most clinicians agree that, because stuttering persons vary enormously, therapy succeeds most when the entire range of behaviors, not just speech, is taken into account. In truth, it isn't really possible for therapy to focus exclusively on speech behavior, although some therapies give that appearance. Regardless of therapeutic approach, the stutterer has feelings about what he is experiencing, just as you do, and these feelings are important, sometimes central, forces in therapy. We have long recognized that therapeutic success or failure is often attributable to the emotional relationship that exists between client and clinician, rather than to specific speech techniques. The relationship is the key. The goodness of the relationship between a client and his clinician is always important, even in therapies that play it down. For example, the fear is sometimes expressed that human engineering approaches to behavioral change might "dehumanize" the clients exposed to them. Although the possibility exists, especially when preset goals and procedures are uniformly applied to different individuals, it may also exist in approaches called humanistic, psychodynamic, or personalistic. If a clinician has sufficient need to dehumanize stutterers he may, unfortunately, do so in any therapy structure. So the client/clinician relationship plays a major role, for good or ill.

At its best, this relationship is a mutually creative one for client and clinician. The word "creative" requires some explanation. All human beings hunger for a satisfying sense of community with others. Through a therapeutic relationship, a client may satisfy this hunger by discovering the human condition and the fluent speaking within himself. In this way the speaker becomes a better instrument for living with others; he *creates self through his relationship with others.*

We encourage you, therefore, to create a therapeutic mood or atmosphere conducive to total growth, a mood that will enhance a therapeutic structure within which there is great *variety* of design, a mood that will enhance interpersonal relationships. This mood would rise above theoretical issues such as whether stuttering is "learned" or "emotional." Obviously all socially significant human behavior is learned, and any behavior important to the individual is linked with emotional life.

We feel that the creative communicative mood is inconsistent with any attitude that derogates a therapy philosophy or a structure that differs from your own. Just as we tolerate and respect the various life styles of our clients, we must also respect the various professional life styles of other clinicians, especially since the whole truth about stuttering is not yet known. Nearly a century ago, William James made the point: "Even prisons and sickrooms have their special revelations. It is enough to ask each of us that he should be faithful to his own opportunities and make the most of his own blessings, without presuming to regulate the rest of the vast field."

## SAMPLING'S OF THE STUTTERER'S WORLD

Stuttering, in one sense, reflects a basic need; it is the need to be fluent, the need for satisfying communication, the need to be in relationship.

It is suicide for me — without my speech. The average guy has his speech — can crack jokes. They do not have to be serious. When you try hard and fight to speak, you can't be flippant and say the things they like to hear. If I could only speak. All I ever get is a kick in the teeth.

For one who is consumed by this need, few other real interests may exist. He swings from one extreme to another; he dreams nightmares of stuttering or has fantasies of fluency; he thinks and feels deeply only about stuttering and fluency; he wants only to be rid of the stuttering and to become fully fluent. Utopia is a place where he speaks forever fluently; if only he could be assured of fluency for the rest of his life, he would be completely happy and would never ask for anything more. All else is less important. Love, respect, trust, esthetic appreciations, relationships with others may be pushed aside as unimportant. The stutterer sees the world darkly through the narrow lens of his stuttering.

There are two approaches you may find helpful in aiding the stutterer to widen his narrow view. The first is to encourage him to *live beyond the stuttering;* this includes living toward one's share of happiness *in spite of* the stuttering. The therapy goal here is to "flood out" the stuttering with satisfying, nonstuttering-related life experiences. Your clinical goal is to move the stutterer from the attitude that "What counts is stuttering" to "What counts is *life.*" All positive characteristics of the stutterer must be given great attention. Each asset of the stutterer must be identified, brought to the fore, highlighted, appreciated fully, praised, and built up all the more. this includes living toward one's helping him to recognize and appreciate that he speaks fluently

most of the time, as is usually the case. It must include identification and supportive recognition of every successful or pleasant (not just fluent) speaking experience. Some stutterers find it helpful to keep a running log and frequency counts of various pleasant speaking and general life experiences which can then be discussed with the clinician or with other stutterers and used as a reference for increasing the frequencies of positively toned experiences. Hobbies, sports, other recreational pursuits, interests in art, readings, sciences, in nature — all are pleasant life experiences which broaden one's perspectives. Therapy will progress more rapidly when the stutterer comes increasingly to see his stuttering in the larger perspective, through the lens of life.

The second way to widen the stutterer's outlook can be described as a movement from "all or nothing" to "little by little." The stutterer of narrow perspective wants fluency — entirely and now, if possible. Anything less is unacceptable and, in fact, is often not even genuinely considered. At the risk of oversimplification, the goal here is to help the stutterer believe that "big oaks from little acorns grow," that greater fluency will follow small gains. You will need plenty of ingenuity to help the stutterer set up a series of steps to small goals, each successively a bit more difficult than the last, and to help the stutterer accept the *importance* of these small steps. It isn't easy for the stutterer to work a step at a time when so much within him cries out for the giant leap.

Maybe it's easier to dream of giant leaps than to take small steps. Nonstuttering adults usually live in safe, orderly, predictable worlds. But the stutterer's world is unpredictable and unmanagable and things happen more often. One of the central purposes of therapy is to neutralize apparent dangers through *knowledge* ("I'm no longer afraid of this thing because I now know something about it") and through *attitude* ("I trust in the goodness of this therapy; I have faith in my ability to learn from experience. I believe that I can improve").

## The Pains of
## Doubt and Guilt

The hunger to speak fluently, the feeling of insecurity connected with stuttering, and the stuttering behavior itself produce many effects, not the least of which are feelings of doubt.

Can I speak when I need to? I never know. I'm never sure. I'm never able to count on saying one word. Never, never, and then I try again. Whose fault is it? It is my fault? If only someone would accept it. Was it all in the cards? How many others are like me? Have I given myself this out — my speech? But

I have a perfectly good mind. Strangely enough, it's my mind that's been killing me. It thinks and picks on every part of my failure. It compares me with people who can do for themselves. It tortures me. How can I use it to deal with problems besides my failure?

Nothing seems worse than constant uncertainty, although in some cases the stutterer may be relieved when he "learns the worst." Doubt is uncomfortable. We try to free ourselves from it, to pass into a state of belief which seems more satisfactory. The stutterer may hold on to his beliefs vigorously, whether they are true or false. Such immovable thought may provide some temporary peace of mind but will not be helpful in the long run. For this reason a stutterer, apprehensive about having to speak publically, might declare that he believes social organizations take advantage of their hard-working members, and refuse to join them; or, believing that others would not be interested in what he has to say, remain silent; or, believing that the clinician must know the answer to his problem, might not actively participate in its solution.[1]

---

[1] The method of fixed beliefs is not peculiar to stutterers; clinicians can become fixed in their own philosophies and methods.

It is paradoxical that the pain of silence may be preferred, perhaps unconsciously, to the possibly greater pain of the unknown ("What *may* happen if I try to speak"). Abandoning the familiar for the unknown always involves risks. The pain of stuttering may also be preferred to the unknown. What is unknown is alien, and the chances of relating to and mastering newer ways of speaking and being are less certain than the old familiar ways. This may be more true in adolescence than in later adulthood. Only after the discomforts have been faced and new competencies and integrations achieved will such disturbances subside. Hope in the possibilities of the new way may diminish the doubts, and more confident actions may reduce the threats, especially if environmental conditions are supportive. When they are not, when the family situation is difficult, for example, the security attached to what is familiar may be clung to tenaciously, though often with continuing, even frightful, doubt and guilt.

It's shameful what I'm doing to my parents. I hurt my mother so badly, I could see the torture in her eyes. It was as if I stabbed a knife in her. I am nothing, a shameful, good for nothing, a being who can only hurt. I lean on others, sapping their strength. What you asked me to do I couldn't do. Anyone else could have done it. Always thinking of myself. I've never made a worthy attempt in my life. I have taken you away from people who could be helped. I have no pity for the good people. I just think of myself. I am no good. I don't deserve the wonderful parents I have. My mother is an angel. So is my father. For years I made my father's life a hell on earth. He didn't deserve it. I still take it out of his hide. I can't go on hurting them, I can't. I'm not as bad as to do that. But I am a sponger. I'm everything bad. I'm not even a person. I have magnified a little thing like a speech defect into a fake bugaboo. What have I done to be made into a monster?

## Fantasy and Frustration

We have observed that stutterers often live by a state of "fixedness," not only in belief but in perception and action; a pervasive fantasy life is one of the results. Sometimes the fantasies are attached to certain categories of people, such as authority figures or women, and become the basis for irrational attitudes toward them. Other kinds of fixed fantasies cause the stutterer to respond excessively or inappropriately to certain situations. Normally, people respond differently to different people and situations. But when a stutterer acts as though every person were out to humiliate him, and when he does this repeatedly, his behavior suggests a fixation or a false belief about others, himself, or the world at large.

The clinician should consequently try to help the stutterer increase his ability to recognize the unique features of others, the things that differentiate people from each other, and help him learn to be interested and excited by the remarkable variety of characteristics people have, even those belonging to a particular group, and including groups of stutterers. Increased sensitivity to the uniquenesses of others will reduce stereotyped responses; and the breakdown of stereotyped thought will help to fragment anxious, fixed attitudes and expectations. Any such reduction will contribute to increased fluency.

### Hostility and Aggression

Not surprisingly, the frustration from imagined or actual rejection can lead to hostile feelings and behaviors. The inability to speak is an inability to live fully. Some express the aggression overtly; others boil within. Even when aggression is turned outward, however, it can fuel self-hatred; more frustration and shame often follow. The sources of frustration are many, but for example, one of our young stuttering friends described how, in the course of a twenty-minute conversation, his father managed to say to him: (1) "Can't you see that I'm just not interested?"

(2) "That's a fault you have, talking about subjects you don't know anything about," (3) "Silence is golden," (4) "A good listener learns a lot of things," and (5) "A constant talker just gives himself away." This may be the briefest manual on "how to make a stutterer." At any rate, this young man had become a complete bore because he acted totally uninterested in whatever anyone else had to say; to his detriment, he had out-fathered father. Fortunately, awareness of the pattern led to a reduction of the behavior and the anger, and to an improvement in social relationships and communicative fulfillment.

Unfortunately, many instances of success are marred by the absence of a sense of fulfillment; most stutterers succeed in a variety of ways, but many can't appreciate the experience. They have not learned to enjoy moments of success sufficiently. They must somehow prove or disprove something, or delimit themselves in some way ("Yes, but I still stutter"). The concept of themselves as successful people may contradict the concept of themselves as stutterers, so they hide the recognition of success, suppress it, forbid its expression.

Our task in such circumstances is several-fold: (1) we must assist the stutterer to express these hidden feelings, get them out into the open; certainly not to force the issue, but to provide an atmosphere of trust so that the client feels freer to share intimate and perhaps forbidden thoughts. Group discussions or role-playing situations may permit this atmosphere to develop. (2) We can help the client evaluate more realistically the purpose of these feelings and the actual effects they may have on behavior. (3) We must support the client's efforts to express his feelings in socially acceptable ways (sports, physical exercise, painting, writing, or other forms of expression) and to discover other ways of reducing the need to have such feelings. (4) We can also help the client increase the number of pleasantly toned speaking situations he enters, beginning with the least threatening ones and working steadily up to more difficult ones. (5) Finally, we can help the client appreciate increasingly every successful moment experienced in both non-speech and speech situations.

## EMOTIONAL DISCOMFORT, ATTITUDES, AND SELF-REGARD

Many stutterers are chronically tense, worried, and uneasy. Clinicians know how important it is to take these things into account in any therapy structure designed to enhance interpersonal relationships. When this chronic condition is severe, it threatens the core of the personality; it may even threaten one's sense of existence. In such a case the word "anxiety" is appropriate. When the condition is milder, however, the term "emotional discomfort" seems better. For most stutterers, the disorder is associated by frequent occurrence with states of emotional discomfort. A major goal of therapy then is to increase the degree of emotional comfort. Many aspects of human activity will require attention to do this, but the attitudes of the individual are one crucial aspect; and where attitudes are concerned the individual's attitude toward himself, his concept of himself, is most important.

### The Stutterer's Self-Concept

Perhaps you have heard people who stutter make statements similar to one or two of these:

(1) I am a stutterer. I am not like other people. I must think differently — because I stutter. (Wendell Johnson)

(2) Had I no hands I would have become a painter. But because I stutter I had to become an actor. (Roger Blin)

(3) When I first heard myself on a tape recorder I wanted to scream, but later I only cried. (junior high school student)

Although declarations like these can be helpful in getting to know clients, the *idea* of self-concept can be vague. Let's define it simply as an individual's view of himself as a person; or, the *me* that one consciously knows, feels, and regards. Questions seeking self-concept might be: "Who am I?" "How do I think?" "What are my evaluations of myself?" "How do I feel about myself?" "How do I compare to others?" "What do others think of me?" and "How do I want others to regard me?' In fact, these questions are often good starting points for discussions.

As Van Riper has observed, the person who says "I am a stutterer" formulates his self-concept in a way that implies compulsive deviancy; such a statement is potent with self-concept. It is like the heroin user saying to himself for the first time, "I am an addict." Self-identification as a member of a minority group is a common expression of self-concept. Following a period of speech frustration and social rejection, the stutterer comes to label himself as such, and to be so labelled by others. It is a sad time.

Many stutterers, in relation to other stutterers, come to avoid what they take to be the displeasure of their company, unlike other groups having members with an impairment in common. One said:

My relations with my fellow stutterers, my companions in sorrow, were hardly congenial, and in fact few people whom I've met have I reacted so violently towards. I saw in them all the atrocities and ugliness that I feared showing so much in myself.

As stutterers learn to regard others who stutter in terms of their total functioning, to appreciate all of their uniquenesses as persons, improvement occurs in their own behaviors, including speech.

Denial of self as a stutterer is another self-deception. Some find it impossible to look at themselves in a mirror while stuttering, or to look into the double-barrelled mirrors of their listener's eyes. They may shut their own eyes, sometimes as a tension reflex, but sometimes to separate themselves from their painful environment. One college student who, by all the evidence, had stuttered for fifteen years, never referred to himself as a stutterer or to his stuttering speech by any common name during the first thirty-two hours of therapy. Any reference to it he couched in circumlocutions: "The thing I do, the little problem, my talking manner, my difficulty, what I'm here for." He finally got secure enough to speak the monstrous word, not explosively as can be the case, but softly, calmly and directly: "I stutter. I am a stutterer. I always have been. It's the truth. Bitter pill to swallow. Off with the armor. So I'm exposed. But I'm ready. Let's go."

The improvement of self-concept is not simple, but it must be attacked, for the stutterer's experience is affected by his self-concept. Our first job is to get to know the client well enough so that we can identify the critical factors, and then work at strengthening some, weakening some, and ignoring others. It is difficult to be explicit about steps to take to improve self-concept. It isn't the same as working with speech behavior, but you should find that fluency increases when self-concept changes. Any of the following events, if they happen frequently, will improve self-concept: (1) Strong, genuine support and faith is shown in the client's ability to improve. (2) Insight about attitudes and feelings is experienced by the client. (3) *Any* acts of accomplishment in speech (including existing degree of fluency) or in nonspeech behavior (such as the conquest of fears or the reduction of speech-avoidance behaviors) are recognized, fully appreciated, and accepted by the stutterer as "mine." Similarly, any genuine *efforts* to succeed, whether successful or not, should be praised (anecdotal records of such efforts might be kept). And (4) any active participation by the client in planning his own therapy. Some clinicians find it helpful to use specific speech assignments suggested by, carried out, and reported on by the stutterer himself. Van Riper provides a large number of practical suggestions along these lines in his chapter of this book. Briefly, then, *any* improvement in *any* activity increases the probability of improving the self-concept and decreasing the stuttering.

While the stutterer may see himself as a stranger in an unpromising land, often enough he takes the opposite tack: people who should be close to him are regarded as strangers, as alien. When you don't know someone very well, it's easier to attribute your own feelings to him, or to assign to him attributes that justify your fears. In a war, one shoots at "enemies" rather than persons. People who are psychologically comfortable do not regard other people as strangers, but then, most people have not experienced the repeated social rejections that older stutterers have, nor have they felt the doubt that follows, the fear, and the growing negative expectancy toward others, with its ever-accumulating derogation to the stutterer's self-concept. Increasingly rewarding social interactions will help. Still, it is difficult to help the stutterer realize he can become a greater and happier person and speaker by becoming a more open, trusting, real self. The goal of being oneself fully is a mighty one, difficult but important. We recall one of the Hasidic stories in which Rabbi Zusya, shortly before his death, says, "In the world to come I shall not be asked, 'Why were you not Moses?' I shall be asked, 'Why were you not Zusya?' "

## FEARFUL EXPECTATIONS

Stuttering has been called an "expectancy disorder," for a major part of the problem is related to negative expectations concerning how others might react to one's efforts to speak. What you expect from any given situation is based on your perception of it. And perception in no small way is determined by motives or needs. The stutterer and non-stutterer alike shape the way they perceive and judge themselves and the world. One attends selectively, reacting to things that confirm and justify expectations, neglecting whatever is contradictory to them. But when we imagine life, we often live what we imagine. No fact exists except as interpreted. If you're optimistic and relaxed, what follows tends to occur as justification. As William James stated, "Believing that life is worth living will help to create the fact."

But believing that life may *not* be worth living will create different facts, and the fearful expectations of stutterers can lead to justifications for their beliefs. For instance, the stutterer sometimes has a peculiar relationship to time, in a variety of speech and social senses. Often he does not seem capable of living life in the present; he lives in a state of expectancy of "what might be," the fearful expectation of failure or listener rejection sweetened only by the hope for happier tomorrows. The capacity to be oneself fully, spontaneously, in the immediate present is reduced. Success can't be truly enjoyed at the moment it occurs because there is always the apprehensive or hopeful look ahead. These self-defeating expectations vary a lot — they may be specific sound or word fears, or a generalized anticipatory discomfort.

Your first job in battling these fears is to identify them, and this can be difficult. First of all, they occur with incredible diversity. Also, fear identification and modification are often resisted or blocked because the cilent is not consciously aware of the sources of his discomfort or because he rationalizes the matter so as to avoid confronting the real issues. He may fear the loss of his self-control or becoming powerless. He may fear the exposure of his "weakness," of being mocked or pitied. Guilt feelings often follow stuttering, and these may be feared themselves. Humiliation or shame intensifies self-doubt and the belief that he is a person of little worth. Anger may follow the frustration or feelings of disapproval, or it may well up before the act of speaking is attempted, further complicating the whole speaking effort. One stutterer said:

> You're right. I'm involuted. I must break out into the world. But it will be hard. I've grown so to fear the world. I see its hardness, its cruelty. The price of failure is tremendous. It means contempt and scorn. I'm sensitive. When I'm not accepted I crumble. Will I have the strength to harden myself and, by battling it all, find myself?

A solution to the negative expectancy problem may be found during a progression of fear confrontations. The client, with the aid of the clinician, develops a hierarchy of his feared situations running from the least to the most greatly feared. One high school stutterer's list, for example, looked like this:

1. Speaking to myself out loud when alone
2. Speaking to pets or animals
3. Speaking to babies or young children
4. Speaking to older children
5. Speaking to my mother
6. Speaking to fellows my age
7. Speaking to girls my age
8. Speaking to my father
9. Speaking to women I don't know
10. Speaking to men I don't know
11. Speaking to store clerks
12. Speaking before a group that knows me
13. Speaking before a group that doesn't know me
14. Speaking on the telephone to a friend
15. Speaking on the telephone to a stranger

Having prepared such a list, the client and clinician work together to set up conditions in which each step can be experienced repeatedly until the situation can be entered without fear. Situations are devised which present progressively greater confrontations, yet which have more chance of success than failure. The experiences will be more successful if they are paired with pleasantly toned associations. Sometimes the situations will require breaking down into more subtle sequences. The approach is explained in more detail by Joseph Wolpe and his followers.

A positive note is struck when the stutterer realizes, and really accepts, that the attitudes of his listeners are frequently determined by his own attitudes toward them; his fantasy eventually becomes his reality. If, upon meeting people, he expects rejection and behaves accordingly, sooner or later he will be rejected. Stutterers provide many examples of self-fulfilling prophesies, and changing the nature of prophesies is an important therapy goal. It is best achieved by reorganizing and reintegrating *all* facets of the stutterer's personality, including a renewal of his faith and trust — in himself and in others. Until this occurs he will continue to expect fearfully and to escape to supposed safety through various avoidances. Desensitization is an important part of this process, but the key to reintegration lies in the reorganization of interpersonal relationships.

## THE CREATION OF SELF THROUGH RELATIONSHIP WITH OTHERS

What does it take to speak? What enhances speech regardless of social or therapeutic setting? Our observations convince us that the following conditions contribute to the stutterer's speaking ability:

1. Whatever helps the client feel freer, share himself, and affect others in socially desirable ways.
2. Whatever helps the client come closer to others, touch them and be touched in any humanizing sense.
3. Whatever helps the client live with greater joyful spontaneity, nonverbally and verbally.
4. Whatever increases his feelings of hope, faith, and trust, in others and in himself.
5. Whatever increases his willingness to risk complete living, the courage to be himself fully.
6. Whatever increases his feelings of personal worth, and his ability to love and be loved.

### From Fear to Courage

How do we help the client take life as he finds it, improving it as he can? Growth is possible only if he has a vision of what things are worth working for and some sense of how easy or difficult they will be to obtain. You play a vital role in helping him see what is possible. Some people are acutely aware of life; they are determined to get the most out of it, in work, play, love, or speaking. It may be that this zest for life can't be taught, but we must believe that it can be learned, perhaps from models, such as clinicians. Only those who are willing to give up a stuttering life, or at least to strive in that direction, will come to know most fully what life is worth. Saying "yes" when everyone else wants you to say "no" shows integrity, a refusal to violate one's emerging identity.

I've always wondered what kind of soldier I would make.

I've always had this image of myself, like a Russian cossack on a white stallion rushing into battle. Do you think I would have been a coward? Now that I've decided to just be myself, maybe I'll find out. It would be nice to be a hero.

Wouldn't you agree that it takes a kind of courage, after failing so often, to try to speak again? Many have buckled under lesser strains. To have people turn away from you, to be left alone, to be alone repeatedly, or always, is something like death, but most stutterers nevertheless return to the fray. Sometimes a stutterer's courage may need help from you, en*courage*ment, but you *can* help most of them, even those with more than average emotional discomfort. When you judge that the emotional problems are too complex for you to deal with, however, or when you yourself feel threatened or repeatedly uncertain about the possible development of dangerous behavior in the stutterer, then referral to a more qualified counseling source is clearly necessary. Most speech clinicians, however, underrate their ability to be helpful in improving a stutterer's emotional behavior, either directly or by working on his speech. Also, the stutterer has a natural tendency to protect himself in the fact of any intervention by another which is truly threatening to his security. Since you can help, and since there is a lack of quali-

fied, available psychotherapists, it is important that you try to improve your ability to deal with the emotional aspects of stutterers' lives.

### A Hope that Is Not Fantasy

Courage and faith will develop only if the client feels *trusting*. You can help him develop this capacity by encouraging him to be open to a widening range of experience, including his own feelings, impulses, and wishes, open to doing what he feels is right and natural, and open to those same rights in others. This self-evolving occurs best when the client is eager to create opportunities that enhance the feeling of hope, or which change false hope, or fantasy, into hope for things that really have a chance of coming true — reality-based hope.

I finally let myself go with this girl. I mean I was just myself, stuttering too. It wasn't easy. But she didn't seem to act any differently so I just went on. We took a walk. It was raining. But everything was soft and quiet and warm. And I spoke to her of how it made me feel. I said that feelings were the most important thing, even sad melancholy ones. And I said maybe these feelings were a block to my getting along with others. She didn't think so at all. I told her about feelings I couldn't even tell my parents or friends — it was a fine experience. Perhaps I can be this way with others. It felt good. Forgetting everything, even myself, but I was really myself, the person I know I am down deep. Could I be this way with my parents too? Maybe I could . . .

Hope is practically an unmentioned topic in the speech pathology literature, but it is an aspect of the therapeutic relationship that is crucial, though not always perceived by either client or clinician. There is no prescription for helping a human being to journey toward greater hope. But the clinician will have to help his client recognize that the problem can potentially be at least diminished. Without this hope it is unlikely that a stutterer would take any action to change existing conditions. He should believe that therapy has a probability of being effective. The clinician's own attitudes, of course, will be critical. The client should feel that the clinician is interested and capable of setting up a relationship that is designed to bring about the change. Hopelessness is chiefly a failure of the imagination. Adult therapy is a relationship in which two or more people imagine the best possibilities, then work for their achievement.

## Self-Reliance and Self-Worth

Creating or inventing oneself means taking responsibility, choosing, risking vulnerability, being able to tolerate the insecurity of growth. The stutterer must develop *self-reliance*. He has to give up self-derogation, self-defeat. He must take responsibility for his speech behavior, for his own therapy program, for dealing with himself more objectively, for following through on developmental tasks. For a stutterer, the idea that he himself might have had an active part in the direction of his life and of his stuttering can be difficult to accept. Even if environmental factors played a part in his development, over time the problem becomes increasingly *his*. As one clinician stated, "He's not guilty because he didn't know better. Now that he knows better he can't keep dodging the responsibility."

Self-reliance means recognizing straightforwardly the part one has played and is still playing in the continuation of the problem and the improved part he *can* play. We must then help the stutterer remove any false fronts, move out of secrecy into openness. But the openness must be genuine. The following note was written by a brilliant college stutterer who was still intellectually defensive:

I am talented in the visual arts — not painting or sculpture — no, in the art of masking — the art of appearance which is disappearance. My stuttering is the mask which keeps me from showing my true face. Of course, masks have their purposes, as do mine. But stuttering's masks are clever and varied — it's hard to unravel the secret behind; even I may not be truly aware of the mask I wear. It's been said that if you are to understand a Rembrandt self-portrait you must study his entire work and his biography. If you are to understand *my* masterpiece, my stuttering, my mask, perhaps you must study me in my entirety. God! Words, words. Another mask?

Feelings of personal worth may be the key to enhancing personal relationships. The clinician tries to help the stutterer see himself as having goodness, as having significant thoughts and feelings to share, as wanting to move toward the humanly good; wanting to share himself with others in close, kind ways, as being likeable and in some relationships lovable, recognizing that his trust in his own ability and potential is usually justified as is his faith in himself and others. As positive self-regard increases, he will open up more, expand his social relationships, enlarge his freedom of expression, extend his spontaneous thoughts and feelings, become more deeply interested in the lives of others, mature.

## BEING A CREATIVE CLINICIAN

To paraphrase an old statement, in stuttering therapy, the cure must be as convincing as the stuttering. That's often a tall order. You can make a good beginning, we think, if you assume the following: (1) No two stutterers are alike. (2) The stutterer himself is the most crucial diagnostician, and perhaps the most crucial clinician. (3) Therapy structures are available along a continuum of different forms. There is not just one set form. (4) The stutterer can contribute actively to the relationship, helping to identify goals and the means for attaining them. And (5) Personal qualities, the clinician's as well as the client's are often crucial, usually more important than the materials or methods used.

Philosophers, writers, psychotherapists, and counseling speech clinicians have long recognized that an accurate and sensitive awareness of another person's feelings, a deep concern for the other person's welfare without efforts to dominate him, and an open, nondefensive authenticity or genuineness will benefit any human interaction. Third Force or humanistic psychologists have stressed the importance of the following characteristics of clinicians: (1) Trustworthy, dependable, or consistent in some deeply important sense. (2) Able to express attitudes of interest, respect, liking, and caring. (3)

Perceives the client as wanting to grow in the most positive sense and as capable of charting much of his own recovery. (4) Shows consonance in what he thinks, says, and feels. (5) In tune with his own feelings and able to express them spontaneously, but with no need to satisfy personal motivations that interfere with therapy. And (6) perceives the client as capable, not only of *being* fully in the present, but as capable of becoming something more than he now is. Perhaps more simply we could say that to fulfill his therapeutic function the clinician must be a person of deeply felt sympathy in his relationship with the client and he must have a genuine and persistent desire to help him.

### Image-Breaking: Permitting Oneself to Be Human

It is remarkable how frequently clinicians, although they might not wish to be so characterized, present to the client the image of a "flawless person." A verbal fly on the clinical wall might give the following report:

This clinician is always punctual and poised; seems to be in calm control of any situation, is always attentive, sympathetic, interested; never gets upset, much less angry; seldom bellylaughs, only smiles modestly at times; apparently has never had any problems since none has ever been mentioned; apparently is never sad, or fatigued, or frustrated for no statements reflecting such conditions have ever been uttered; in addition, this clinician is a confident speaker.

The therapy relationship is unreal if, over a long period of time, the clinician never expresses annoyance, skepticism, or similar feeling. There are limits of course to such expressions of authentic humanness, but to be rigidly consistent or unreally perfect will eventually erode the relationship. As one stutterer complained,

I needed him to serve as a kind of model, not only someone I could count on but someone I could admire and maybe even try to be like. I finally realized that nobody could be perfect, but he seemed to want me to think that he was. He just wasn't natural. I got suspicious. He never made a mistake, even when it was a tough problem. I don't have a ghost of a chance of being anything like that. Didn't want to anyway. I got turned off.

There is a strong likelihood that a person will not fully open up about himself to others unless he believes that the audience, social or therapeutic, is genuinely of good will. Self-disclosures occur in settings of trust and love. With love, or of deep liking if you will, one can let the other know him more fully. No change of real interpersonal significance is possible otherwise. In a trusting relationship, the client is in a mood to risk, a mood the recovering stutterer must experience if he is to unmask himself and work toward individual human authenticity. The clinician, too, must occasionally risk. Real change can occur when the clinician who has, probably unwittingly, presented an image of perfection to his client finally relieves himself of the burden of having nothing but beautiful feelings.

Interpersonal growth in stuttering therapy occurs in different ways: (1) by improving the skills of speech behavior, (2) by satisfying basic needs, (3) by modifying or removing anxiety, fears or apprehension, (4) by having self-fulfilling or self-actualizing experiences, (5) by emotional release or catharsis, and (6) by self-understanding. Stutterers vary a lot and some will improve most with a domineering clinician, others with more easy-going ones. All therapies will result in improvement, if only by suggestion, if the client has confidence in the clinician. The clinician himself will often induce this confidence, regardless of the therapeutic model, by his own self-confidence, his vitality, sincerity, ability, and interest. He may also bring it about, at least for a while, through gimmickry, showmanship, or pure arrogance, but such instances, fortunately, are rare.

May we suggest, especially to the self-actualizing clinician, that from day to day or when in doubt, do what you yourself consider humanly kind and important. In so doing, you will rarely be far from responding helpfully to the needs of a stuttering person.

ALBERT MURPHY

# The Clinician and Therapy

Stuttering is more than just stumbling over words; it can be stumbling over self as well. Therapy too is more than the routine application of techniques; its effectiveness depends on what you put into it. So the stutterer's problems grow out of who he is, and therapy grows out of who you are. In this chapter we'll look closely at the therapy process and if you'll also look closely at yourself you may be able to *vitalize* whatever procedures you use.

## THE NATURE OF THERAPY

What is therapy? Certainly it is change, change in behavior, in attitudes, in circumstances or desires, but not all change is therapy. Stutterers change with the passage of time, through self-treatment or parental treatment, and in reaction to situations they encounter. These changes may be improvements, or they may not, and the total effect is probably random. Therapy, however, isn't random; it's a special kind of change, with distinct characteristics. There are at least five qualities that distinguish therapy from other kinds of change: First of all, therapeutic change is focussed on a target, so that it has direction. Second, it's more rapid than the change produced by unsystematic efforts. Third, it's consistently constructive. Fourth, the changes occurring in therapy are more stable and long-lasting. And fifth, the pace of therapeutic change is steady. These five characteristics are not distinctly separate, they interact with one another to give therapeutic change a special quality that's hard to sum up but is nonetheless distinct from other kinds of change.

Some activities look like therapy and may even be called therapy but aren't. Poorly conducted sensitivity groups, for example, may introduce so many destructive elements that they offset any gains. Some procedures done in the name of therapy for stutterers produce temporary improvements but lack stability. Others produce long-lasting changes but in the wrong direction by producing new and undesirable accessory features or a manner of speaking that is more objectionable than the way the client talked before treatment.

Other activities don't look like therapy but share some of its characteristics. Through constructive interaction with a friend, for example, a stutterer may become more fluent, more self-confident, and less withdrawing. But therapy should do these things and others more efficiently.

The changes produced by therapy may have profound effects, far beyond the speech pattern. The way a person speaks is a product of many different things, of learned behaviors, of feelings, conscious and unconscious, of personality structure, and of the nervous system's efficiency. Your therapeutic impact is aimed at all of these things, so that when you enable the stutterer to make changes in his behavior, you change much more than behavior. If you can be aware of this broad context and alert to some of the wider effects your efforts may have, you'll be a better clinician.

Being alert to the effects you're having will make you wonder about how much control you have, or should have, over the process of therapy. The amount of control depends on what you think you're doing or should do. Do you see yourself as doing something *to* the stutterer — making him do certain things that will cure him? If that's *all* you see, your therapy may be cold, detached, and manipulative. You may even shift from controlling the process of therapy to controlling the client. A more moderate degree of direct management would include giving strong suggestions for activities and outlining procedures for the client to follow. On the other hand, do you see yourself as providing opportunities for the stutterer to achieve understanding and thus to alter his behavior? This is a more indirect approach. If you're too indirect, the client will be forced into taking nearly all the initiative. He'll be his own therapist, even while working with you, and you'll have little control over his activity.

The control you exert should probably vary considerably at different stages in therapy, with the age and sophistication of the stutterer, and with the techniques you feel qualified to use. The important point is that you'll probably be more effective and adaptable if you're aware of how much control you're exerting and what effects different amounts of control may have.

Your therapeutic approach will depend on your own concept of therapy, the training you've had, the models you've observed, and the personality of the stutterer. Whatever you do, you'll be working with a complex person, made up of drives and energies in a dynamic equilibrium, with functions that stabilize and change. You're inserting a new factor into this composite — a special kind of interaction between you and the client. The nature of that interaction is the essence of therapy.

## PERSONAL ATTRIBUTES OF THE CLINICIAN

Personal attributes can have a lot to do with successful therapy. In fact, some clinicians rely on them so heavily they neglect their technical competence. Others try to ignore personal factors in an effort to be objective and scientific. But impersonal therapy is a mechanistic and sterile process, like painting by numbers.

The most effective clinician develops himself and learns about himself at the same time that he acquires the technical skills and knowledge of his profession. All of us can improve as creative clinicians if we become more aware of the existence and importance of certain aspects of our personalities. We hope this chapter will help you learn more about characteristics that are particularly important for working with stutterers.

## General Attitudes

The way you work with stutterers will reflect a number of attitudes you have developed. For instance, how do you view therapy? Do you see it as a great leap from a defective to a normal way of speaking? Or do you see it as a series of discrete steps from one level to another? Actually, neither view is very accurate. Therapy involves simultaneous movement along several interactive dimensions. Progress along each is relative to the others, not absolute. One of these dimensions is fluency, clearly a fluctuating activity, measurable only in relative terms. We want the client to become more fluent by reducing the number of his disruptions and by teaching him better ways to manage any disfluencies that do occur. And we want these changes to occur in a greater variety of situations. At the same time, other important dimensions of behavior — attitudes, feelings, understandings, assumptions, and concepts — may also need attention. The interaction of these dimensions, including fluency, must be considered. For instance, a desirable change in feelings may cause a decrease in fluency, at least temporarily. Therapy is consequently a dy-

namic process, not a sudden jump, or even a step-by-step change from "defective" to "normal." If you look at therapy as a series of categories, you'll over-simplify and compartmentalize your interactions with the client. You'll fall into the trap most stutterers are already caught in — you'll just want to see him quit stuttering for good. Success, in that case, is limited to the absolute sense of the word — it no longer has relative degrees along different dimensions. As you begin to sense therapy as a flow along selected but connected channels, you'll become a more effective influence.

Therapy can also be seen as continual problem solving. Far from being incompatible with the idea that therapy is a dynamic process, the problem-solving approach implements this view. If you maintain the problem-solving attitude, it's possible to remain flexible, adaptable, and responsive to the varying needs of the client. You can then freely alter your procedures and goals as evidence indicates the necessity to do so — not because you have failed in an earlier approach but because you're adjusting to what the situation demands. Of course, you shouldn't make such changes whimsically, but flexibility does help you to avoid being a slave to the "rules" of therapy. For instance, it's a general rule to encourage the stutterer to become his own therapist. In one sense of the word, you *must* do this if he's going to modify his speech over a long enough period so that the improved pattern will become automatic. At some point in the therapeutic process, however, you have to provide support and direction. This was well illustrated in an intensive program for stutterers during the summer of 1971. One of the stutterers had, through the years, developed a fierce independence. At first, the clinician worked on the assumption that this independence could be used, and he let the client make a great many of the decisions about therapy. As therapy evolved, however, it became apparent that the young man had reached a point where he needed considerable support and direction. The clinician then altered his approach and started making more of the decisions. This didn't mean the original approach was wrong or that the clinician had failed; the approach had simply served its purpose for the time being. Changes in the client dictated a change of approach, and it was made.

The problem-solving attitude also gives you a basis for analyzing why anticipated successes may not have occurred. You can look not only at the techniques and procedures you've been using but also re-evaluate your original goals, then make readjustments in either.

One plus for the problem-solving attitude is what it can do for you. Do you "lose patience" quite easily? What do you "lose"? You may become irritated, frustrated, and experience feelings of impending failure. But you haven't run out of something you should have more of. You just stopped looking at the situation as a problem to be solved and inserted some irrelevant and interfering emotions. If you can achieve this attitude in therapy with stutterers, you'll find it possible to go on looking for different ways to resolve the difficulty. If the client doesn't do what you thought he would, you assume that the appropriate methods haven't been found and you go on looking for or creating them rather than becoming exasperated. If finally you run out of solutions you accept this for the time being and go on to a different aspect of therapy. This may be mildly frustrating, but it may also leave you with the nagging feeling that there is a solution you have yet to discover, and that's a good thing.

### Specific Attitudes

One thing that will have great impact on your therapy is *your concept of the client.* You should already have a favorable feeling toward clients or you wouldn't be a speech clinician. You can develop and expand this feeling by placing the client first in your time and attention when you're doing therapy or preparing for it. And if he's that important to you, you'll listen to him and find him worthwhile, not because he does or doesn't have certain qualities but because he's a human being. If you can think about him and others in this way, you'll respect him for his unique personal identity. And if you respect his humanity, you'll have faith in his ability to move in the direction of improved communication. You'll see your job as helping to *release* this ability. The more you respect him and his ability to improve the easier it will be to let him become independent from you. Don't let the client become a satisfying object of dependence to you. If you do, you'll resist the ending of therapy and your client's final improvement. You should rejoice at his success — and in yours as a clinician who can encourage his independence at an appropriate time.

Another trait of the better clinician is *tolerance of uncertainty*. One of the most obvious and pervasive characteristics of life is the incompleteness of what we know for sure. Yet we must function in the midst of this ignorance. Stuttering provides us with considerable uncertainty, and some clinicians are uncomfortable working with stutterers for this reason. Not only is there doubt about the disorder's source, but the results of therapy are often uncertain because fluency is so variable and for a host of other reasons. Also, therapy may have delayed effects. So, you must be able to accept considerable uncertainty if you want to work with reasonable confidence. It's most important that you don't allow your discomfort with the uncertainty to cause you to give up too fast on a procedure or activity.

We have noted already that therapy involves change. Some clinicians may be uncomfortable because nothing in therapy appears settled. In the stutterer's speech, in his reactions, in situations and different environments, in the choice of procedures there is always variability and fluctuation. You can never settle into a comfortable, steady movement from here to there in your therapy. Examine your *reactions to rapid or erratic change*. If it makes you uncomfortable or if you fight it, perhaps you should work toward accepting it in order to reduce your discomfort.

You may also be dismayed by the *complexity or diversity of stuttering* and its therapy. There are so many aspects that are active, that need almost your full-time attention. You may feel as if you're juggling seven balls in the air at once, and the constant effort to keep track of them results in frustration, anxiety, and feelings of impending failure, or at best, an uncertainty that you may not be getting anywhere. Can you handle complexity, or is it an area for you to work on?

Your basic attitude toward these conditions — uncertainty, change, complexity, diversity — is based on another orientation of considerable importance. What are the *sources of your own security?* Many people equate security with stability, but you can feel secure with movement and change. If you can develop a dynamic security, you'll have a confidence that is constructive and helpful in therapeutic interaction. And if therapy for stutterers is to improve, it too must change.

### Specific Awarenesses

Other attributes that are helpful in therapy with stutterers are best identified as awarenesses. They vary in breadth, intensity, and specificity, but all can add strength and effectiveness to your therapy.

*The Significance of your work.*

Your awareness of the significance of your work as a speech clinician provides a context for all that you do and has particular importance for stuttering. If you're not a stutterer and don't know any stutterers well, you may not appreciate how deeply they are affected by their difficulty in speaking. Because of this social importance of being able to talk accurately and fluently, speech therapy has an unusual significance.

The need to communicate is so pervasive and intense that any interference with it threatens the individual in a way that is hard for him to manage. When communication is imperiled by distortion or distraction, fears and anxieties mount and may themselves interfere with communication. Why is communication so important? One reason may be that it increases our *awareness of being alive.* We have many sources for this awareness, for example, sensory impact. A sudden and complete loss of hearing can cause profound depression far beyond the fact that the individual has difficulty receiving information. We live in a barrage of noise, and without it the sense of being alive is diminished. Talking is just the expressive side of the same coin, and when the ability to talk is impaired in any degree, our sense of being alive is diminished. The same thing happens when the people we can communicate with deeply and easily are far away from us. A stutterer also has a barrier to his communication, and consequently feels a loss of self.

Communication is also important because *it reduces our sense of being alone.* Although we would not want to eliminate this feeling entirely, since some aspects of our nature are best served by solitude and isolation, our whole society is geared to help us reduce the feeling of being alone. One of the primary drives for learning speech comes from the child's awareness that he can substitute words for physical contact to reduce his aloneness. Later in life, we use phrases of greeting to continue this verbal reaching out.

Of course, we also communicate to *express ourselves* — to share what we feel and know, not for the good of others but for the satisfaction we get from sharing the wonder and excitement of an insight, a bit of knowledge, an experience or understanding that is meaningful and important to us. Language crystalizes an experience and makes it even more our own by letting us share it. We express our longings, hopes, and fears to release the anxieties they engender and to clarify our understanding and to realize our potential. Most importantly, we express our love and concern for others, for the only way to know we are loved is to express love for someone else. The person who can't do so is most miserable because no matter how much positive feeling others may direct toward him he never *knows* he is accepted and loved. Here the stutterer feels most keenly the effects of his halting speech.

We also *reach out* when we communicate — to explore and experience as a way of expanding, enhancing, and enlarging the self. Language and speech enormously widen our range of experiences. Through communication our individual environments expand to include the environments of all those we talk with, and all those *they* talk with, and so on to include all of the experiences of humanity. A person who has deficiencies in his speech is limited much like someone who has physical deficiencies that limit the range of his movements. In most cases, however, a speech deficiency can be reduced or removed by appropriate therapy. As a result the person becomes more effective, develops a greater complexity, and becomes more nearly complete.

Since the ability to talk satisfies such deep psychological needs, we are each obligated to become as good clinicians as possible. As a clinician, you reach deeply into the stutterer. So you must understand your own needs to do your job with insight and impact.

## Why are you a speech clinician?

Your work should contribute to your own individuality if it's going to be more than just something you do to earn money. What can speech therapy do for *you?* A personal answer to this question will make you more effective.

There are a number of ways *your work can contribute to your development as an individual.* It extends the dimensions of your participation in life. You're not sitting on the sidelines, you interact intimately with people, responding to some of their basic needs. Over a period of years you will have developed a series of constructive human relationships, and this adds depth to your own being. Then, because language is basic to the vital elements which make us human beings, your intimate contact with others and their problems improves your own self-understanding. Finally, being a clinician helps you develop because you participate in problem solving without being sucked into the destructive vortex of the problems themselves.

*The work you do is complex* enough to challenge you for a lifetime. You never solve the last problem; you continue to have new worlds to explore. At the same time, speech therapy has some simplicities, some routine, and some immediate rewards, without which the unending complexities might wear you down. This kind of balance can be exceptionally rewarding and is not characteristic of many ways of earning a living.

If you become more aware of these reasons for being in the profession, and see how they apply to you personally, you're on the way to becoming "consciously dedicated." Unlike compulsive dedication, which drives a person against his will, conscious dedication is being aware of the personally meaningful rewards that come from your activities. It makes you want to do your job where it's most challenging, in deprived rural or urban situations, for instance, and still maintain your enthusiasm.

But watch out. Some immediate satisfactions end up having negative effects. If you think of yourself in therapy as an oracle, a fount of all wisdom, or if you want to manipulate people, you may end up in trouble. If through therapy your clients become dependent on you, the dependency will become a burden you'll want to be rid of as the years go on.

## Self-Awareness

You need to be aware of your behavior as you do therapy. You have to learn how to monitor your behavior and to do this without being self-conscious, or feeling discomfort or anxiety. You need to scrutinize your behavior and see which aspects of it are facilitating and which might be inhibiting the progress of your client. You must also know when you're making judgments and what your judgments are based on. This means separating facts from assumptions and not being dogmatic, rigid, or routine as you apply techniques. Monitoring yourself can be as simple as noting that you are beginning too many sentences with "well" or calling your client by name repeatedly. Maybe you are interrupting him so frequently that it interferes with the interaction. Or you may follow the same kind of therapeutic pattern with different clients without thinking enough about whether it is appropriate for the person. As we become more experienced, all of us are inclined to repeat whatever has been successful. We have to climb out of these ruts, and a good way to do it is to keep checking yourself on it. Make *that* a habit. Otherwise, you can become stereotyped and progressively less effective in therapy.

## CLINICAL SENSITIVITY

The awarenesses we have described contribute significantly to your clinical sensitivity, but further development of this important attribute is always desirable. Clinical sensitivity doesn't mean having a frail ego that is easily hurt. And it doesn't mean feeling sorry for the handicapped or someone in trouble. Clinical sensitivity is a heightened awareness of the client's needs, an awareness that makes it possible to make objective judgments about therapy. Part of this sensitivity is being able to reduce your personal identification with the problem and maintain a kind of distance between yourself and the client's difficulty, even though you may develop a closeness for the client himself. You set yourself aside so that you are not pulled down into the client's misery, so that you can respond constructively to his problems.

You can increase your sensitivity by observing yourself, because sensitivity is a reactiveness within you. Try to learn the source of your feelings and reactions. How much of your response, for instance, is due to empathy? How much is due to the stimulation of your own similar problems? As you observe yourself, while still oriented to the other person and his needs, you will find your sensitivity increasing.

## MATURITY

People who are more mature are probably better clinicians because they can be more reactive to the client's needs without letting their own egos get in the way. They're better able to apply their professional knowledge and skills. Maturity is particularly important with stutterers because the complexities of therapy put great demands on our understanding, creativity, and adaptability.

Maturity is reflected in *the way you behave*, but there's no absolute standard of mature behavior. And you don't just become mature and then stop changing.

There will be fluctuations from time to time and situation to situation. Nevertheless it's possible to distinguish behavior that is more mature from behavior that's less mature, according to certain criteria.

What makes behavior mature? Some of it has to do with *your philosophy of living*. All of the decisions you make are affected by your ideas about the meaning of why you exist. This doesn't mean you have to have a "deep" or well organized or even verbalized philosophy, but people who keep asking "Who am I?" "What am I?" "What kind of universe am I in?" "What is the meaning of my thoughts and actions?" probably exhibit more mature behavior. Less mature people either reject the idea of needing to think about the meaning of life, or they are completely settled and have all the answers. It's more mature to be aware of the need for a continual development in understanding, of new insights and attitudes which modify and expand your ideas. And this development continues throughout life. You don't suddenly "become mature." This awareness of the need for growth must be applied to your professional life if you're going to be the best kind of clinician for stutterers.

Greater maturity also means *accepting reality as it is* rather than the way you think it ought to be. Look at driving a car, for example. Your ability to stay alive while driving is based on how well you can see reality for what it is and react to what needs to be done rather than to irrelevant factors such as the way you "feel." For instance, if the car ahead signals a turn and you continue to drive at the same speed on the assumption that it's going to complete the turn and get out of your way, this is naive. The driver may not turn, or he may turn only part of the way. Then you're in trouble. Similarly, if your judgment of what is happening in therapy is clouded by what you want or expect to happen, you're short-changing your clients.

At the same time, you should be aware that *you can influence reality*. To accept it as fixed is not a mature attitude either. By its very intent, therapy is designed to change things, so your conviction that you can influence reality is vital. The mature person is always aware that he has some influence, but he knows his limitations.

*Being able to accept responsibility* is another sign of maturity. Some people even equate maturity with this trait. In the clinic your ability to make judgments, and to accept the results without being disorganized, is an important measure of your maturity. Just deciding to help others indicates that you're willing to accept responsibility. But don't take on too much. It isn't necessary for you to accept responsibility for the total life of your clients. Some judgment about how much responsibility you can and should accept is necessary.

The more mature person is *goal directed* too. He's aware of and moves toward distant goals. This certainly applies to the treatment of stuttering. If you're looking for the quick cure of stuttering, you'll probably use one of the techniques that bring temporary fluency. Being able to move systematically and persistently toward distant goals is essential since therapy with stutterers takes a considerable length of time. At the same time, the mature person doesn't hold these distant goals in the forefront of his consciousness all the time. They should be set out as clearly as possible, and the client should be on the road toward reaching them, but most of the clinician's time is spent attending to the immediate needs of therapy and to attaining intermediate objectives. So when we say that you should be goal directed, we mean that the general direction of therapy should be determined by general, or distant, goals, while more specific activities will be determined by short-term goals.

Your maturity, then, can be seen in the way you evaluate yourself and your work. You should have faith in your decisions, realistic expectations, and a reasonably broad perspective about the problems you're trying to solve. Each of these characteristics shows up in the way you work with stutterers.

## ROLE ACCEPTANCE

To become a successful clinician, you have to accept various roles. You will have to be a supervisor, initiator, parent substitute, an information source, a monitor, and many other things. At times you have to be demanding and stimulating, at other times passive and receptive. Some of these roles will be out of line with your own inclinations or life style. The better therapists learn how to extend themselves, how to vary their roles. They aren't limited to the roles that appeal to them personally. In order to adapt to the needs of different stutterers at different times, you have to have many roles you can accept.

About this time you may be saying "How can I ever expect to do all this? How do I become all these things and acquire these attributes?" The answer is simple (but the acquisition isn't). You change the same way your clients do. Set up goals, experience attempts to improve, evaluate yourself and try again in light of the evaluation. Focus on the things that seem most difficult, since they'll take the most time and effort to attain. At the same time, you should become aware of the attributes that you already have or that come to you easily and use them as effectively as possible. Through this kind of process you will develop as a person and increase your skill as a clinician.

* * * * * * * * * * * * * * * * *

We hope this book has given you some understanding of stuttering and some suggestions for how to solve this many faceted problem. We have presented the sequence of evaluation and assessment; the identification of the details of stuttering; the reduction of emotions that intrude on speech; the modification of unwanted behaviors; and the transfer and maintenance of new ways of communicating. At the same time we have described the problems of motivation; the altering of feelings, attitudes, and beliefs that influence speech; and the importance of knowing about the nature of therapy and yourself as a human being. But this isn't enough. How you put the parts together is critical. But the most important ingredient in successful therapy will be your own unique and personal addition. If you have the kind of optimism that sees in each stutterer his tremendous potential for becoming whole and free, every session will be an extension of the best that is in you. Add to this a sense of vibrant living, and therapy becomes life at its highest. So take everything we have said, add yourself to it, and go on from there. Whatever you do, don't stop here!

STANLEY AINSWORTH